WHY CAN'T I LOSE WEIGHT?

By the same author:

Low Blood Sugar
Diets to Help Diabetes
Diets to Help Migraine
Why Am I So Tired?
Recipes for Health: Low Blood Sugar (with Maggie Budd)

Why Can't I Lose Weight?

**Is Your Weight Gain
a Symptom of a Hidden Health Problem?**

MARTIN L BUDD N.D., D.O.

Thorsons

Thorsons
An Imprint of HarperCollins*Publishers*
77–85 Fulham Palace Road,
Hammersmith, London W6 8JB

The Thorsons website address is: www.thorsons.com

and *Thorsons*
are trademarks of HarperCollins*Publishers* Limited

Published by Thorsons 2002

1 3 5 7 9 10 8 6 4 2

A catalogue record for this book
is available from the British Library

ISBN 0 00 712065 6

Printed and bound in Great Britain by
Martins the Printers Ltd, Berwick upon Tweed

Contents

PART THREE: HELPING YOURSELF AND THOSE
YOU CARE ABOUT

While the author of this work has made every effort to ensure that the information contained in this book is as accurate and up to date as possible at the time of publication, medical and pharmaceutical knowledge is constantly changing and the application of it to particular circumstances depends on many factors. Therefore it is recommended that readers always consult a qualified health specialist for individual advice. This book should not be used as an alternative to seeking specialist medical advice, which should be sought before any action is taken. The author and publishers cannot be held responsible for any errors and omissions that may be found in the text, or any actions that may be taken by a reader as a result of any reliance on the information contained in the text, which is taken entirely at the reader's own risk.

Acknowledgements

Once more, my love and thanks must go to my wife Maggie for her typing and computer skills.

Apologies to our dog Peppa, for all those promised, but missed, Sunday walks.

Artwork by my brother Simon Budd.

How to Use This Book

This book has been written to draw attention to the many reasons for weight increase. For the frustrated dieters who just cannot lose weight, it will be a great relief to know that diets and exercises are not always the answer. So often, the huge number of books written describing special diets and exercise programmes fail to mention the third component for successful weight reduction: our metabolic efficiency and status.

The topics discussed in this book do not include life-threatening diseases, but mild functional disorders that can often be reversed and solved.

Readers will notice a common theme to the many health problems that are described in this book. When your metabolism is faulty, your overweight is never the only symptom. The symptoms that accompany your extra weight should serve as useful clues to the underlying health problems. For example:

Overweight with fatigue	May be caused by hypothyroidism (see Chapter 9), low blood sugar (Chapter 2) or candidiasis (Chapter 5).

Overweight with a monthly pattern	May be caused by PMS or a hormone (progesterone/oestrogen) imbalance (Chapter 8).
Overweight following antibiotics	May be caused by an enzyme deficiency (Chapter 7), 'leaky gut' or food intolerance (Chapter 6).
Overweight with indigestion	May be candidiasis, hypothyroidism, enzyme deficiency or food intolerance.

Identifying the Causes

A good first step is to list your symptoms. I always request a symptom list from my patients. When this is presented, they are often astonished and embarrassed at the variety and amount of their symptoms.

Many health problems show a characteristic symptom-picture or profile. However, a word of warning: there may be two or more reasons why your metabolism is contributing to your overweight. Yes, you may have candida overgrowth and food intolerances, but you may also be suffering the effects of a low thyroid.

This book is not a self-treatment manual, but rather a review of the many health factors contributing to overweight. Hopefully readers will be able to identify with some of the case histories included in the book.

Sometimes a slight change in your diet, say to include more raw foods or reduced carbohydrates, can have a dramatic effect on your weight. Simply by reversing lunch and dinner so the smaller meal is at the end of the day can have an impact on your weight. Drinking extra water can also be a valuable aid to weight loss.

However, certain disorders that influence our weight may need to be diagnosed and treated by a professional. Laboratory testing is sometimes essential, and only an experienced doctor or naturopath can prescribe the appropriate dietary supplements.

Response Time

We are encouraged to believe that with the help of 'wonder' products and special diets we should lose 5–7 lb (2.3–3.2 kg) in seven days. This type of 'crash' dieting is temporary and unrealistic. A good weekly maximum for weight loss is 2 lb (0.9 kg). However, it is worth remembering that metabolic weight increase can only be permanently reduced when the underlying causes are reduced and removed. Many practitioners who treat chronic metabolic overweight refer to the 'one-month, one-year' rule. This proposes that the time to diagnose, treat and obtain weight loss could equate to a month per year of symptoms. So if you have been overweight for six years, it may be six months before the causes are identified, treated and a predictable response is beginning to reduce your weight. This time factor is demonstrated in many of the case histories described in this book.

For those readers who are able to establish the causes of their overweight, whether as a result of their own efforts or with professional help, their success brings with it a welcome bonus. In addition to weight loss, they will certainly experience general health improvement. Physically and mentally they will feel an increased vitality and greater sense of well-being. With the help of this book, you should be able to overcome the obstacles to weight-loss you have faced, and be healthier and more in control of your life.

Part One

Questions

Introduction

Why Can't I Lose Weight?

If you have picked up this book, you have probably had a problem, in spite of your best efforts, at losing weight and/or keeping it off successfully.

If you have found that following special diets and exercise programmes only results in temporary weight loss, with the weight then piling back on faster than you lost it, or if you find that you are putting on weight even though you are not eating more or leading a less active lifestyle then in the past, then your excess weight will *not* be your only symptom. Other symptoms may include fatigue, indigestion, muscle pain and stiffness, poor concentration, depression and a galaxy of similar health issues.

Metabolic Imbalances

When excess weight is caused by ill-health of this kind (sometimes termed 'metabolic obesity'), low-calorie diets and exercise programmes will only provide short-term results, if that. If your metabolism and body chemistry are depressed, deficient or imbalanced, the causes need to be identified and treated before any programme of weight loss can begin to work.

There are those who see overweight as simply a direct result of overeating. However, I have seen patients increase their weight even when following an 800-calorie a day diet!

This book offers a step-by-step programme to show you how to identify the cause or causes of your overweight. Diagnosis does not always rely on elaborate and expensive laboratory testing. Many aspects of our metabolism can be measured and assessed quite simply at home.

However, it may be necessary to use blood tests to assess your thyroid function, blood fats, sugar and insulin levels. All these procedures will be explained, and their value assessed, in this book. We will also discuss the general health benefits of a healthy diet, nutritional supplements and exercise programmes.

A single diet that can help anyone lose weight does not exist. There is evidence to show that our family history, our food, the work we do, the way we handle stress, our personality and even our blood group can all influence our body weight.

My portfolio of diet-sheets for my patients includes 32 different programmes, and I am still designing new ones. We are all metabolically unique. Learning more about our imbalances and deficiencies can be the key to satisfactory weight loss.

CHAPTER ONE

What Is Overweight?

What exactly does it mean to be overweight, and how can excess weight be defined? Given that our genes, our lifestyle and occupation, our body-type and our health history are all uniquely different, just how do we know when we are overweight?

There is certainly no shortage of words and phrases in the English language to define overweight. A good thesaurus usually includes 25–30 synonyms, and there are possibly an equal number of euphemisms.

This breadth of definition regarding overweight can be attributed, in part, to cultural and national differences. In many countries, excess weight in women is seen as an attractive, sought-after attribute and a yardstick for femininity and potential fertility. In the US, on the other hand, near-anorexic models are seen by many as representing the ideal female shape. In Western Europe and America, overweight is usually associated with ill-health, laziness, loss of pride and self-discipline. Role models and media celebrities are strongly influenced by this concept that 'the thinner, the better'. People who remain slim are seen as healthy, largely successful and in charge of their lives. Our appearance, as much as our personality, knowledge and skills, has become an important element in career advancement, relationships and success in every field.

With the existing differences, culturally and nationally, when defining overweight, could it be argued that the 40% of women in the UK who are officially 'overweight', are in fact of average or normal weight, and the other 60% more right defined as 'underweight'?

Some years ago, a colleague of mine visited friends in the US and stayed with a family in a country area. He weighs around 11 stone (154 lb/70 kg) and he is 6 ft tall. After his first week he telephoned me to tell me how kind and solicitous his hosts were. They frequently offered him a chair, and were forever asking him how he was. It was only after he was asked what treatment he was receiving that the reasons for their concern became apparent. Essentially, they had assumed, because of his appearance, that he was suffering from terminal cancer. He of course reassured his hosts that he was fine and well. Upon his return to England he explained to me that the average weight of the American males that he'd met was 15–18 stones (210–252 lb/95–114 kg), so they saw him as being severely underweight and therefore very ill. He was a normal, ideal weight, yet in their world he was seen as a very sick man.

Weight Charts

We are all familiar with the height/weight charts found in books and journals. These usually provide the recommended weights for different heights, male and female. Sometimes specific weights are shown as 'ideal', or a 'normal' range is offered.

I often wonder who devises these charts, because the recommended ideal weights tend to vary from chart to chart. Add to this the existing differences in our world (culturally and nationally) when defining overweight, could it be argued that the 40% of women in the UK who are officially 'overweight', are in fact normal?

Let's take a look at ways to assess your own ideal weight and potential fat burden – and also to ask the question: when is weight 'normal' and just how do genetics, body-type, age, lifestyle and diet influence your optimum weight?

Ideal Weight?

Although an obsession with our weight can be unhealthy and self-defeating, we all would like to know what constitutes our ideal weight. How we look and how we feel are obviously very important to most of us, but when planning any type of weight-loss programme, we need to have some idea of our healthy weight target.

Up to very recently, the majority of height/weight charts used by dietitians and doctors were based on figures put together many years ago. These were derived from data and weight associated with 'lowest death rates', as utilized by life insurance companies to assess risks and premiums, etc. Medical dictionaries printed within the last six years still tend to include such outdated and unreliable tables. These usually sub-divide each height level into three frame sizes: small, medium, and large. The only problem is, the 'ideal' weight varies by as much as 36 lb (16 kg), depending on one's frame.

These weight variables for a given height are excessive and confusing. As you cannot define your 'frame size' accurately, such wide variations in 'desirable weights' really give you no useful information at all. (The basis of such subdivisions is the assumed weight variations of the human skeleton's 206 bones. In reality, the weight difference of a small person's skeleton and a large person's skeleton of similar height is only around 12 lb/6 kg.)

Old Fashioned Height/Weight Tables

Desirable weight in pounds and kilograms (in indoor clothing), ages 25 and over

MEN

Height (in shoes)			Small frame		Medium frame		Large frame	
ft	in	cm	lb	kg	lb	kg	lb	kg
5	2	157.5	112–120	50.8–54.4	118–129	53.5–58.5	126–141	57.2–64
5	3	160	115–123	52.2–55.8	121–133	54.9–60.3	129–144	58.5–65.3
4	4	162.6	118–126	53.5–57.2	124–136	56.2–61.7	132–148	59.9–67.1
5	5	165.1	121–129	54.9–58.5	127–139	57.6–63	135–152	61.2–68.9
5	6	167.6	124–133	56.2–60.3	130–143	59–64.9	138–156	62.6–70.8
5	7	170.2	128–137	58.1–62.1	134–147	60.8–66.7	142–161	64.4–73
5	8	172.7	132–141	59.9–64	138–152	62.6–68.9	147–166	66.7–75.3
5	9	175.3	136–145	61.7–65.8	142–156	64.4–70.8	151–170	68.5–77.1
5	10	177.8	140–150	63.5–68	146–160	66.2–72.6	155–174	70.3–78.9
5	11	180.3	144–154	65.3–69.9	150–165	68–74.8	159–179	72.1–81.2
6	0	182.9	148–158	67.1–71.7	154–170	69.9–77.1	164–184	74.4–83.5
6	1	185.4	152–162	68.9–73.5	158–175	71.7–79.4	168–189	76.2–85.7
6	2	188	156–167	70.8–75.7	162–180	73.5–81.6	173–194	78.5–88
6	3	190.5	160–171	72.6–77.6	167–185	75.7–83.5	178–199	80.7–90.3
6	4	193	164–175	74.4–79.4	172–190	78.1–86.2	182–204	82.7–92.5

WOMEN

Height (in shoes)			Small frame		Medium frame		Large frame	
ft	in	cm	lb	kg	lb	kg	lb	kg
4	10	147.3	92–98	41.7–44.5	96–107	43.5–48.5	104–119	47.2–54
4	11	149.9	94–101	42.6–45.8	98–110	44.5–49.9	106–122	48.1–55.3
5	0	152.4	96–104	43.5–47.2	101–113	45.8–51.3	109–125	49.4–56.7
5	1	154.9	99–107	44.9–48.5	104–116	47.2–52.6	112–128	50.8–58.1
5	2	157.5	102–110	46.3–49.9	107–119	48.5–54	115–131	52.2–59.4
5	3	160	105–113	47.6–51.3	110–122	49.9–55.3	118–134	53.5–60.8
5	4	162.6	108–116	49–52.6	113–126	51.3–57.2	121–138	54.9–62.6
5	5	165.1	111–119	50.3–54	116–130	49–59	125–142	49.4–64.4
5	6	167.6	114–123	51.7–55.8	120–135	54.4–61.2	129–146	58.5–66.2
5	7	170.2	118–127	53.5–57.6	124–139	56.2–63	133–150	60.3–68
5	8	172.7	122–131	55.3–59.4	128–143	58.1–64.9	137–154	62.1–69.9
5	9	175.3	126–135	57.2–61.2	132–147	59.9–66.7	141–158	64–71.7
5	10	177.8	130–140	59–63.5	136–151	61.7–68.5	145–163	65.8–73.9
5	11	180.3	134–144	60.8–65.3	140–155	63.5–70.3	149–168	67.6–76.2
6	0	182.9	138–148	62.6–67.1	144–159	65.3–72.1	153–173	69.4–78.5

Mosby's Dictionary Fourth Edition 1994

(To obtain weights for adults aged between 18–25, subtract 1 lb for each year under 25)

Somatotypes

Another method of grouping body-types is known as *Somatotypes*. While this classification cannot be relied upon totally, certain characteristics of the three types can provide interesting and useful clues to account for people's different responses to specific diets and weight-loss programmes.

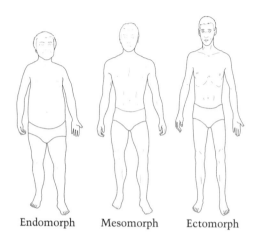

Endomorph   Mesomorph   Ectomorph

Based on physical characteristics, the three main somatotypes are:

- Ectomorph or aesthetic
- Mesomorph or athletic
- Endomorph or pyknic

Although there are those who exactly fit into one of these sub-groups, many of us have a body type that includes a mix of two different types.

ECTOMORPHS
These are slim individuals with highly developed nervous systems and poorly developed digestive systems. They do not usually have much interest in food and drink, and often maintain a healthy weight throughout their lives. Ectomorphs rarely need to look at diet books.

MESOMORPHS
These are predominantly muscular individuals possessing a heavy, hard physique (mainly muscle weight). Mesomorphs tend to gain

weight at middle-age. They usually benefit from a low-carbohydrate/ high-protein diet, coupled with plenty of exercise.

ENDOMORPHS

These individuals are characterized by a soft, rounded frame with a large trunk and thighs and tapering legs. They tend to accumulate fat easily and have a well-developed digestive system. Pure endo-morphs can have great difficulty maintaining a healthy weight. They usually benefit from a low-carbohydrate diet.

As I have said, most of us represent a bit of a mix of these three groups. However, I am sure many readers will know friends or loved ones who appear to fit perfectly into one of the groups.

Not surprisingly, particular groups tend to run in families, and although your somatotype classification should not be seen as a major hurdle to successful weight loss, there is little doubt that those who are predominantly endomorphic can face more of a battle when it comes to weight loss than their ectomorph and mesomorph counterparts.

Now let's look at the more up-to-date and reliable procedures for assessing your ideal weight.

Body Mass Index (BMI)

The Body Mass Index (BMI) is currently seen as an effective method of assessing your ideal weight. It is calculated using an equation that also takes height into account, making it more precise than relying only on scales. The BMI does not allow for variations in bone, fat, muscle and organ weight, meaning that an athletic individual and a desk worker who never exercises can have similar BMIs. This is because fat weighs less than non-fat lean muscle.

The Body Mass Index (BMI) is calculated as follows:

Your weight in kilograms (1 lb = 2.2 kg) divided by your height (in metres) squared.

For example, if you weigh 160 lb (72.7 kg) and your height is 1.6 m (5 ft 4 in), your BMI will be 72.7 ÷ 2.56, to give you the BMI of 28.

Excess weight will increase your BMI. The ranges are as follows:

Weight	BMI
Normal weight	20–25
Overweight	25–30
Seriously overweight	30–40
Dangerously overweight	40+

Some authors recommend different scales for the two sexes, however, as women's BMIs are only very slightly lower than for men, the above ranges can apply to both sexes.

Body Mass Index

		ft in	5'6"	5'7"	5'8"	5'9"	5'10"	5'11"	6'0"	6'1"	6'2"	6'3"
		cms	168	170	173	175	178	180	183	185	188	190
lbs	*stns/lbs*	*kgs*										
88	6/4	40	14	14	13	13	13	12	12	12	11	11
90	6/6	41	15	14	14	13	13	13	12	12	11	11
93	6/9	42	15	15	14	14	13	13	13	12	12	11
95	6/11	43	15	15	14	14	14	13	13	12	12	12
97	6/13	44	16	15	15	14	14	14	13	13	12	12
99	7/1	45	16	16	15	15	14	14	13	13	13	12
101	7/3	46	16	16	15	15	15	14	14	13	13	13
104	7/6	47	17	16	16	15	15	15	14	14	13	13
106	7/8	48	17	17	16	16	15	15	14	14	14	13
108	7/10	49	17	17	16	16	15	15	15	14	14	13
110	7/12	50	18	17	17	16	16	15	15	14	14	14
112	8/0	51	18	18	17	17	16	16	15	15	14	14
115	8/3	52	18	18	17	17	16	16	16	15	15	14
117	8/5	53	19	18	18	17	17	16	16	15	15	15
119	8/7	54	19	19	18	18	17	17	16	16	15	15
121	8/9	55	19	19	18	18	17	17	16	16	15	15
123	8/11	56	20	19	19	18	18	17	17	16	16	15

lbs	stns/lbs	kgs	5'6" 168	5'7" 170	5'8" 173	5'9" 175	5'10" 178	5'11" 180	6'0" 183	6'1" 185	6'2" 188	6'3" 190
126	9/0	57	20	20	19	19	18	18	17	17	16	16
128	9/2	58	21	20	19	19	18	18	17	17	16	16
130	9/4	59	21	20	20	19	19	18	18	18	17	16
132	9/6	60	21	21	20	20	19	19	18	18	17	16
135	9/9	61	22	21	20	20	19	19	18	18	17	17
137	9/11	62	22	21	21	20	20	19	19	19	18	17
139	9/13	63	22	22	21	21	20	19	19	19	18	17
141	10/1	64	23	22	21	21	20	20	19	19	18	17
143	10/3	65	23	22	22	21	21	20	19	19	18	18
146	10/6	66	23	23	22	22	21	20	20	19	19	18
148	10/8	67	24	23	22	22	21	21	20	20	19	18
150	10/10	68	24	24	23	22	21	21	20	20	19	19
152	10/12	69	24	24	23	23	22	21	21	20	19	19
154	11/0	70	25	24	23	23	22	22	21	21	20	19
157	11/3	71	25	25	24	23	22	22	21	21	20	20
159	11/5	72	26	25	24	24	23	22	21	21	20	20
161	11/7	73	26	25	24	24	23	23	22	21	21	20
163	11/9	74	26	26	25	24	23	23	22	22	21	20
165	11/11	75	27	26	25	24	24	23	22	22	21	21
168	12/0	76	27	26	25	25	24	23	23	22	21	21
170	12/2	77	27	27	26	25	24	24	23	22	22	21
172	12/4	78	28	27	26	25	25	24	23	23	22	21
174	12/6	79	28	27	26	26	25	24	24	23	22	22
176	12/8	80	28	28	27	26	25	25	24	23	22	22
179	12/11	81	29	28	27	26	26	25	24	24	23	22
181	12/13	82	29	28	27	27	26	25	24	24	23	23
183	13/1	83	29	29	28	27	26	26	25	24	23	23
185	13/3	84	30	29	28	27	27	26	25	24	24	23
187	13/5	85	30	29	28	28	27	26	25	25	24	23
190	13/8	86	30	30	29	28	27	27	26	25	24	24
192	13/10	87	31	30	29	28	27	27	26	25	25	24
194	13/12	88	31	30	29	29	28	27	26	25	25	24
196	14/0	89	32	31	30	29	28	27	27	26	25	24
198	14/2	90	32	31	30	29	28	28	27	26	25	24

BMI Electronic Scales

These can be purchased at many retailers and specialist medical suppliers. They calculate weight and BMI values, and usually include an 'Ideal Weight Indicator'. They have a capacity to weigh up to 146 kg (23 stone/322 lb) and retail at under £50.

Resting Metabolic Rate (RMR)

This defines our resting calorific profile, or daily calorific requirements, and indicates the amount of heat we lose as we are active throughout the day (i.e. that occurs with the metabolic process). Although this sounds rather complicated, a simple self-assessment test can be done as follows:

If you are under 30, multiply your weight (in kilograms) by 14.7, then add 500.

If you are over 30, multiply your weight (in kilograms) by 8.7, then add 830.

Exercise, temperature changes, digestive efficiency and your hormone balance can all increase your calorific need by increasing your metabolic rate. To arrive at a figure for your daily calorific intake, you will have to adjust the figure of your RMR as follows:

If you have an active job and do regular exercise	Multiply your RMR by 2
If you do sedentary work and take only a little exercise	Multiply your RMR by 1.7
If you do sedentary work and take no exercise	Multiply your RMR by 1.4

Examples

Susan   Age 29   Weight 60 kg (132 lb)

A desk worker doing no exercise, Susan requires 1,935 calories daily
(60 × 14.7 + 500 × 1.4 = 1,935).

Tom   Age 49   Weight 88 kg (194 lb)

An active manual worker, Tom exercises daily and requires 3,191
calories a day (88 × 8.7 + 830 × 2 = 3,191).

You can use this guide to work out your metabolic calorific requirements. It is easy to see how exercise makes such a difference to your
daily calorie needs.

Lean Body Weight or Mass (LBW or LBM)

This represents the ratio of muscle and bone to body fat. The fat-free
parts of the body (also termed the 'lean body compartment'), have
been established for healthy individuals at 82–90% for men and
75–85% for women. Women, therefore, do tend to carry a higher
percentage of fat than men. The total ideal body fat percentages
(BFPs) for healthy individuals are as follows:

Men   Between 10% and 21% of total body weight
Women   Between 20% and 31% of total body weight

It is this fat percentage, or mass, that is the chief concern of the
overweight. The object of dieting is to lose body fat while maintaining muscle quality and bone strength.

Body Fat Measurement
The evaluation of body fat percentage has never been an exact science. The traditional method involves the use of callipers on various

parts of the body. A simple 'pinch' test on yourself can be a revealing method to assess excess fat. Using your thumb and index finger, pinch the fleshy skin at the back of your upper arm. If your finger and thumb are more than 2 cm (3/4 in) apart when you squeeze, then the chances are that you are overweight.

Fortunately, there is a more accurate and precise method to measure your body fat status.

Body Fat Monitor Scales

Similar to bathroom scales, these useful machines provide readings of body fat to the nearest 200 gm (0.5 lb). Your height and weight need to be keyed in before standing on the scales. The percentage of fat is assessed by the use of what is called 'electronic resistance measurement' or 'bioelectrical impedance analysis'. Although many sports clubs and gyms provide these machines, they can be purchased from retailers and medical supply specialists for as little as £50.

The ideal body-fat percentages according to age are as follows:

Age	Males	Females
10–30	10–18%	20–25%
31–40	13–19%	21–27%
41–50	14–20%	22–28%
51–60	16–20%	22–30%
60+	17–21%	22–31%

Weight and Food

As we have seen, assessing whether we are truly overweight or not can be complex. And an important variable that must be factored in is how we *feel*.

To return to the perennial question 'Why don't I lose weight when I eat less food?', there are many who still hold the erroneous view that overweight people must be either greedy or lazy. This mistaken view is often 'supported' by the statement that 'no one put on weight in the wartime concentration camps'. This is a mistaken and callous analogy, as neither the desperately ill and dying inmates of those camps nor the modern victims of anorexia nervosa should be used as examples of successful slimming.

In fact, there is evidence that the survivors of concentration camps, when released, frequently became obese upon resuming their normal lifestyle and diet. Their weight-loss in the camp involved muscle-loss as a result of the appalling camp-life and diet, and their metabolism was so altered that the majority subsequently became overweight. This points to what is often the true culprit behind an inability to lose weight even when taking in less food: a problem with an altered metabolism.

As far back as 1919, researchers found that subjects who became slim on a 1,500-calorie-a-day diet were soon overweight again when they returned to a normal diet. Simply eating less may not be the route to weight loss for all.

When talking to my patients, I quite often compare their body's use of food to a car's use of fuel. We all have a good idea how far our car will run on a full tank of fuel. This assumes an average speed of 45–50 mph. If we are allowed perhaps 10 gallons instead of 15 gallons, we can still cover the same total mileage, but we must travel more slowly, with less use of the throttle. So, instead of averaging perhaps 45–50 mph, we may have to average 30–35 mph. In other words, by reducing the engine revs and using less fuel, we are able to travel the same distance.

In a similar manner, a reduced-calorie diet tends to depress our resting metabolism so that we can manage to live and work without the need to use reserve fuel. In simple terms, the body becomes used to a lower-calorie fuel supply and does not need to utilize fat and carbohydrate reserves for fuel; hence the weight tends to plateau. It may take several weeks for the metabolism to 'get the message' and for regular weight loss to occur. This trend, however, soon stops as the resting metabolism adjusts to the new lower food intake.

Unfortunately, with this lower resting metabolism in place, if you go back to a normal diet, you will put weight back on rapidly.

The influence of a reduced-calorie diet on our resting metabolism can cause a 45% depression of the metabolic rate.

With intermittent, repeated bouts of low-calorie dieting, the resting metabolism can fall to such an extent that the metabolism can 'match' the reduced food intake to the point where no further weight loss is achieved – and you hit a plateau for good and all. This can be frustrating and disheartening, and the subsequent return to a normal diet leads to a rapid increase to your original weight, or above it.

Weight-loss Strategy

My strategy to lose weight comprises three components:

1 **Health assessment**
Chapters 2–9 provide information on the health problems that can lead to overweight. These are listed under the headings of symptoms, self-assessment, and diagnosis and treatment.

2 **Your diet**
What type of diet will work best for you? Many factors should influence your choice. Should you follow a high- or low-carbohydrate diet, a high- or low-fat diet, a high- or low-protein diet? Such questions can only be answered with an understanding of your metabolic type, your health history and current health status, your lifestyle, personality and occupation.

3 **Exercise**
Below, we take a closer look at this one.

Exercise

The whole argument for or against the value of exercising to aid weight loss revolves around the balance between energy use or expenditure (e.g. work, exercise) and food and drink intake (e.g. calories, diet balance and type).

When high-calorie diets (e.g. 5,000 calories per day) match our energy requirements (for example if we are endurance athletes – marathon runners, long-distance cyclists, etc.), our weight usually remains at a constant, healthy level. Manual workers (including ground workers, lumberjacks, farm labourers and hod carriers, etc.) can consume 5,000–7,000 calories daily without weight increase. So a high level of activity, whether at sport or work, calls for an appropriate calorie intake that may be 2–3 times the average food consumption. The food is converted to energy instead of being stored by the body as excess weight.

A very high-calorie diet can be justified for reasons other than high energy needs. One obvious example is the increased food required to maintain an optimal body temperature. The explorer Sir Ranulph Fiennes consumed over 5,000 calories each day on his North Pole trek. He was pulling a sledge weighing over 500 lb (228 kg) in unbelievably low temperatures. In spite of his high-calorie diet, his energy output plus the energy required to maintain his body warmth and remain alive caused him to utilize around 11,000 calories daily. Not surprisingly, he lost weight, including muscle wastage.

I am not suggesting that exercise alone will control your weight, unless of course you plan to emulate Sir Ranulph! Nevertheless, it is wise not to become too obsessed just with what you eat. You also need to look at your body's other metabolic needs when planning a successful weight-loss programme.

Exercise – The Case Against
The opponents of exercise as an effective method of weight control have offered two chief arguments:

1   Exercise tends to increase the appetite, so that any benefits achieved by burning off more calories are offset by the increased food intake.
2   The increased metabolic rate and subsequent 'calorie-use' with exercise are minimal compared with that achieved by low-calorie diets.

Exercise – The Case For
My own view is that exercise can have a radical and lasting effect on excess weight. References are available to confirm that inactivity closely parallels weight gain.

Even obese schoolchildren frequently follow lower-calorie diets than their normal-weight, more active peers – yet in spite of this, remain obese.

Exercise and the Brain

Some exercise critics have argued that, as the brain and our total skeletal muscles have similar oxygen requirements, controlled anxiety or any accelerated brain activity could in theory help us lose weight as efficiently as exercise – in spite of the fact that the brain weighs approximately 3.0 lb (1.0 kg), while our skeletal muscle weighs around 80–90 lb (36–41 kg) for an adult male.

However, the ratio of brain and muscle calorie use becomes very different with vigorous exercise. Under such conditions, the oxygen/energy requirements of the brain remain virtually unchanged, while the energy generated by skeletal muscles can increase by 100–120%.

Top athletes can almost double their calorific intake with 2–3 hours' vigorous training daily, without any weight increase.

Unfortunately, few of us are 'top' athletes. So how does exercise influence the average person's metabolism?

Changes to Your Metabolism

With whole-body exercises such as swimming, running, cycling or rowing, many people can increase their metabolic rate by 8 or 10 fold for a sustained period.

Significantly, this type of vigorous exercise will maintain a raised metabolic rate for 12–15 hours after the exercise is over.

Those involved in sedentary work frequently find that the delicate balance between food intake and energy expenditure is not achieved. Essentially, too much fuel (food) and not enough activity becomes the routine, resulting in a gradual weight increase.

Data has shown that those who are required in their work to be regularly active do not find it difficult to maintain an optimum weight. In addition, it has been demonstrated that regular, light exercise can actually serve to depress the appetite and subsequent food intake.

In addition to the three components of my weight loss programme (health assessment, your diet, and the value of exercise), I shall also describe specific supplements that can safely be taken to improve health and to reduce weight.

Part Two

Answers

Sugar and Your Weight

In this chapter we will take a look at low blood sugar (hypoglycaemia) and high blood sugar (diabetes). Either can make you put on weight, and can lead to other health problems, some of which can be quite severe.

Low Blood Sugar and Your Weight

Symptoms

Mental-emotional symptoms	Anxiety, depression, irritability, forgetfulness, poor concentration, panic feelings, phobias, agoraphobia, hyperactivity
Digestive symptoms	Indigestion, bloating, stomach cramps, food cravings, allergies, stomach ulcers and gastritis
Nervous system	Headaches, neuralgias, epilepsy, vertigo, tinnitus

General symptoms   Fatigue, overweight, PMS, joint
and muscle pain, low libido,
fainting, muscular stiffness,
blurred vision, migraine, cold
extremities, sweating and
excessive yawning

When you scan this list of symptoms, you will realize that low blood sugar is not a rare complaint.

Causes

Hypoglycaemia is chiefly caused by a high-sugar diet. Such a diet upsets the delicate sugar-insulin balance and encourages the body to release more insulin to achieve the correct level of blood sugar. This excessive insulin (or hyperinsulinism) can cause chronic low blood sugar levels.

When the blood sugar falls, we do not need sugar. If we take sugar we are stressing what is an already overworked blood sugar control system. The only satisfactory answer lies in careful low-sugar eating with the support of specific supplements and nutrients.

Is Low Blood Sugar Contributing to Your Weight?
Complete the following questionnaire to see if you are suffering from hypoglycaemia. For questions 1–7 give yourself 0 for every 'No', 5 for 'Sometimes', 10 for 'Often'.

1 Do you feel tired and thick-headed when you wake, even after a full 6–8 hours of sleep?
2 Do you experience a sugar craving mid-morning or mid-afternoon?
3 Do you awaken between 3 and 4 a.m. feeling nervous and panicky with sweating or a rapid pulse?

4   Do you have regular sugar/chocolate cravings?

5   If a meal is delayed or missed, do you become moody and nervous?

6   Do you experience a real energy surge when you eat?

7   Is your energy unpredictable and changeable throughout the day?

8   Is there anyone with Type II (maturity-onset) diabetes in your family?

Yes: 5
No: 0

YOUR SCORE

0–20	Low blood sugar is an unlikely factor with your weight
20–40	Low blood sugar could be a factor with your weight
40–75	Low blood sugar is very likely to be a factor with your weight

For many people, everything to do with hypoglycaemia or low blood sugar is confusing. My first book, *Low Blood Sugar* (1981), was written to offer some answers to the questions that puzzled my patients. Some of their most common questions are:

1   How can I have low blood sugar when I eat plenty of sugar?

2   Why is my recommended diet almost identical to my father's diet, when he has high blood sugar (diabetes)?

3   I have been tested many times by my doctor, but my blood sugar is always normal.

4   We are told that we all receive body messages which we should obey, yet when I feel weak and crave sugar why do you tell me it's the worst food I could eat?

5   Diabetes runs in several generations in my family, so why do I seem to suffer the opposite condition?

Answers

1 Hypoglycaemia is chiefly caused by a high sugar diet. Such a diet upsets the delicate sugar-insulin balance and encourages the body to release more insulin in order to achieve the correct level of blood sugar. This excessive insulin or hyperinsulinism can cause chronic low blood sugar.

2 Diabetics need to restrict the sugar in their diet because they cannot produce sufficient insulin to maintain a normal healthy blood sugar level.

3 This is known as 'random' testing and is virtually useless as an accurate guide to low blood sugar. A six-hour glucose tolerance test (which I shall describe later), is an altogether more accurate and reliable test.

4 When the blood sugar falls, we do not need sugar. If we take sugar we are stressing an overworked blood sugar control system. The only satisfactory answer lies in careful low sugar eating with the support of specific supplements and nutrients.

5 Although low blood sugar and diabetes may appear to be opposite conditions, they belong to the same family of conditions. Low blood sugar frequently precedes late onset diabetes. Many of my patients with low blood sugar have a diabetic parent or grandparent.

Low Blood Sugar – The Effects on Weight

Low blood sugar can lead to excess weight for four reasons:

1 Sugar-craving is a well-defined symptom of low blood sugar, and any food rich in sugar is high in calories.

2 Fluctuations in blood sugar levels can cause frequent hunger pangs, which are only relieved by constantly overeating.

3 The stress to the body produced by hypoglycaemia causes large amounts of potassium to be lost in the urine, mainly as

a result of adrenal exhaustion. (The adrenal depletion that results from any form of long-term stress highlights a 'design fault' in our metabolism. Adrenaline is released in response to stress, but it is also released when our blood sugar falls too low or too quickly.) The potassium loss and resulting sodium (salt) retention can cause tissue waterlogging (oedema) and overweight.

4   In hypoglycaemia there is often an excess of blood insulin. Insulin is the only body hormone that promotes the storage of fuel (food). For this reason, it is often termed the 'fattening hormone'. It converts and stores carbohydrate to glycogen, and fat to triglycerides in the liver and muscles.

The combination of high starch and sugar craving, fluid retention and raised fat storage is bad news for any dieter.

Testing for Hypoglycaemia

The Glucose Tolerance Test
The GTT is a six-hour test, and it is seen as a reliable method to identify low blood sugar. It is only a valid test for diagnosing hypo-glycaemia, however, if the following conditions are met:

1   The preparation and sample timings are standardized for each test.
2   The glucose dosage of 50 gm is the same for each test.
3   The patient is relaxed during the six hours.
4   The patient's diet has not changed prior to the test.

TEST PROCEDURE
The patient is requested to fast on water only for 14 hours prior to attending for the test. No food or drink is allowed during the test (except water) and smoking is not permitted. As activity can reduce the blood sugar level, rest is encouraged during the test.

During the course of the test, seven small blood samples are taken from the veins of the arm. (Glucose meters, designed to measure blood sugar levels from a tiny sample of blood, can be used if reliable).

The first sample shows the patient's 'fasting' level of sugar in the blood. The patient is then given 50 gm (approx 2 oz) of soluble glucose to drink, half an hour later. The remainder of the test involves taking blood samples at regular intervals. If, for example, the first blood sample was taken at 9.15, and the soluble glucose taken at 9.30, the rest of the test would go as follows:

Sample 2   10 a.m.
Sample 3   10.30 a.m.
Sample 4   11.30 a.m.
Sample 5   12.30 p.m.
Sample 6   2.00 p.m.
Sample 7   3.30 p.m.

GTT RESULTS

This valuable test can establish a diagnosis of either hypoglycaemia or diabetes. Although the established medical view holds that hypoglycaemia is a rare condition, increasing evidence points to the contrary.

The symptoms that arise during the test are also useful in making a diagnosis. Frequently the patient's chief symptoms (such as headache, dizziness, mood swings, etc.) will occur during the six-hour test. This provides a useful confirmation that a fall in the blood sugar can produce these symptoms.

When patients have a chronic long-term set of symptoms, such as migraine or asthma, their symptoms do not always reproduce during a six-hour test. I have seen GTT results showing profound falls in the blood sugar, yet the patient has not experienced any adverse symptoms during the test time. There is an explanation for this apparent non-reaction to the blood sugar fluctuations during the six-hour GTT:

1 Occasionally there is delayed response to the test, and some patients experience a symptom reaction on the following day.
2 If the symptoms have been around for several years, the patient's metabolism may have developed a glandular compensation to the effects of sudden swings in the blood sugar. This would tend to mask any symptoms, even when sudden changes in the blood sugar level are evident in the results.

Other tests used to diagnose hypoglycaemia include the Glucose-Insulin Tolerance Test and the Serum Mineral Profile. The Glucose-Insulin Tolerance Test involves measuring both the blood insulin and the blood glucose levels over, again, a six-hour test period. Although diagnostically useful it is an expensive test, and I find in my practice that the standard GTT provides sufficient information. The Serum Mineral Profile measures the blood levels for calcium, magnesium, zinc, copper, iron, chromium and manganese.

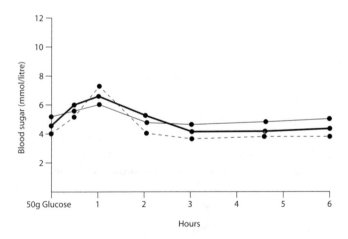

Fig 1. *Normal Blood Sugar – normal curves*
The curves are for healthy individuals. The fasting test (the first reading) varies, but at no time during the six hours does the blood sugar fall much below the fasting level.

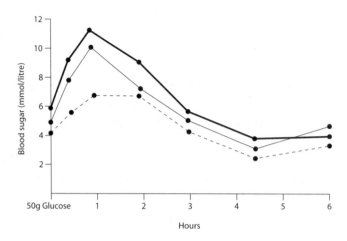

Fig 2. Reactive Hypoglycaemia – typical curves
All the signs of true reactive hypoglycaemia can be seen here. The rapid absorption and rise in blood sugar; followed by the hypoglycaemic 'low' point reached after four hours, and the partial recovery by the six-hour test.

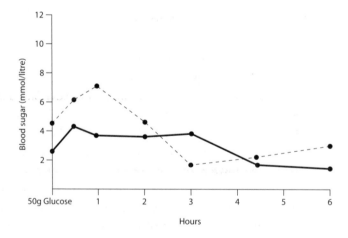

Fig 3. Reactive Hypoglycaemia – severe curves
Often a low fasting level with a further drop into very low readings. Patients with symptoms during the test are usually found to have this type of severe curve.

Treating Low Blood Sugar

There are certain requirements to be met if a diet for hypoglycaemia is to be effective.

These are as follows:

1 The total carbohydrate consumption must be reduced, and refined carbohydrates avoided absolutely.
2 There should be 5–6 small meals daily.
3 The fat and protein components of the diet need to be spread over the day, and included in each meal.
4 The total calorific value of the day's food should not be in excess of 2,500 calories.
5 An early breakfast and late supper are essential.
6 'Stimulants' such as cola drinks, caffeine, chocolate, alcohol and tobacco must be avoided.

Jill's Story

Consultation

When I tell my patients that I suspect hypoglycaemia (low blood sugar) to be their problem, a frequent reply is 'That's impossible, I eat plenty of sugar.' Jill was a case in point. Very overweight at 230 lb (104 kg) and 5 ft 8 in (173 cm) tall – her BMI was therefore 35 and well into the 'obese' range – Jill was 34 years of age and very anxious, very tired and very lonely. She worked as a junior school teacher and had been seriously overweight for 12 years. She always managed to lose weight on diets, sometimes as much as 2 stone, but usually replaced the weight at a faster rate than she'd lost it. She admitted that her sugar cravings were her undoing.

Diet
Jill's diet was as follows:

On rising	1 cup of black coffee with 2 teaspoons of sugar
Breakfast	1 slice of toast with marmalade, 2 coffees
11 a.m.	Coffee with 3–4 biscuits
Lunch	Usually a jacket potato or cheese sandwich with a coffee
3 p.m.	Coffee and 3–4 biscuits
5 p.m.	Coffee and chocolate bar
Dinner 8 p.m.	Usually pizza or pasta dish or Chinese or Indian take-away
	Fruit or yoghurt, 2–3 glasses of red wine
Evening	Chocolates and coffee

The diet did not include fish or red meat. Poultry was the chief protein source. Jill did not smoke, but she ate approximately 1 pound of chocolates as evening snacks each week.

Symptoms

Jill's symptoms included swollen ankles, stiff and painful knees, lower back and neck (particularly on rising, when she also felt sluggish and tired). She experienced bouts of breathlessness, heartburn and frequent migraine-like headaches. If she did not eat for two or three hours, she felt shaky, dizzy and could not stop yawning.

Jill's non-physical symptoms included irritability (she was feared by many of her pupils for her quick temper), anxiety, loss of self-esteem and self-confidence, poor short-term memory and depression. Unfortunately Jill lived alone and rarely saw her parents. She had not been involved with a partner for over three years, and her loneliness fuelled her low self-esteem and her desire for sugar-rich comfort snacks.

Diagnosis

I decided, after discussing her problem and her poor diet, that Jill needed to be checked for low blood sugar. All her symptoms, including her sugar-craving, non-stop yawning and her state of mind, suggested a diagnosis of adrenal exhaustion and low blood sugar. I therefore requested a Serum Mineral Profile and a GTT.

Jill's GTT Results

9.15 a.m.	Fasting Level	(1)	4.6 mmol/L
9.30 a.m.	50 gm Glucose		
10.00 a.m.		(2)	6.3 mmol/L
10.30 a.m.		(3)	7.5 mmol/L
11.30 a.m.		(4)	2.8 mmol/L
12.30 p.m.		(5)	1.9 mmol/L
2.00 p.m.		(6)	2.4 mmol/L
3.30 p.m.		(7)	3.5 mmol/L

The GTT results confirmed reactive hypoglycaemia. Within two hours of drinking the glucose, Jill's blood glucose was at 2.8 mmol/L (anything below 3 mmol/L can cause symptoms). Another hour later, the levels of glucose had fallen to 1.9 and Jill was feeling shaky and anxious, with palpitations and sweating. For her metabolism this was a crisis situation, and adrenaline was released to begin to raise the blood sugar level. Even so, after the full six hours Jill's blood sugar had not normalized, showing a level of 3.5. It needs to be remembered that:

a) 50 gm of glucose is a small amount of sugar.
b) Jill was relaxed and rested during the test.
c) Under work or stress conditions, her response to the glucose and the adrenal compensation would be more severe.

The adrenal system has many functions, and overuse of any one activity can depress and exhaust the others. Jill's diet – high in caffeine, sugar and chocolate – was causing glucose surges in her blood, with resulting hypoglycaemia and adrenal compensation.

Her adrenal system was being overworked, so her inability to handle stress, her anxiety and the joint stiffness and pain were probably caused by the resulting adrenal exhaustion.

The Serum Mineral Profile also revealed that Jill had low levels of magnesium, zinc and chromium.

Treatment

I considered that the priority for Jill's treatment was to normalize her blood sugar level. In achieving this, her sugar-craving and many other symptoms would very likely improve. A diet and exercise programme could then follow to reduce her weight. I prescribed my standard Low Blood Sugar Diet (see pages 46–48). This is a low-sugar, low-refined carbohydrate, reduced-calorie plan with small frequent meals to stabilize the blood sugar.

I encouraged Jill to have fish at least twice weekly. In addition to the diet I prescribed GTF Complex™ (see page 51). This includes the minerals that she was deficient in, plus a specific adrenal support.

Follow-up

It is rare to request a follow-up GTT. When a patient has avoided sugar for several weeks, taking 50 gm of glucose can cause a very unwelcome response which can also be diagnostically ambiguous. The symptom-relief is normally sufficient proof of progress. Certainly, within three months Jill was looking and feeling better. Her mood was also better, and her anxiety and depression were occasional rather than daily symptoms. Although she had yet to give priority to weight loss, her blood sugar diet had in fact helped her to lose 10 lb (6 kg) in the initial three months of treatment.

After Jill had followed the Low Blood Sugar diet for four months, I advised her to have a fresh fruit day every fourth day (see Chapter 7) and, with her improved energy, to consider starting regular exercise. Jill chose to cycle to work each day and to swim 2–3 times each week.

We last met nine months after her initial consultation. Jill looked well and happy. Her weight had fallen to 182 lb (82 kg), giving her a BMI of just under 28. She needed to lose another 24 lb (11 kg), but as she had averaged a weight loss of 1–1½ lb (¾ kg) each week over the previous nine months, I saw no reason why Jill should not reach her target within another four months.

Jill was like so many other frustrated weight-watchers, whose excess weight and fatigue can lead to apathy and loss of self-esteem. Such symptoms can establish a vicious circle of overweight, snack and reward eating, with more overweight.

I believe that often the best way to break such a vicious circle is to give priority to improving the patient's wellbeing and physical and mental energy. When this has been achieved, any weight loss programme becomes easier to follow and, ultimately, successful.

The Glycaemic Index

All carbohydrates metabolize into sugar in the blood stream. The Glycaemic Index gives an indication of the speed at which the carbohydrates convert. Foods with a high G/I listing, cause a rapid rise in the blood sugar, this signals the pancreas to release insulin. Foods with a low G/I listing, release glucose from carbohydrates slowly into the bloodstream, providing essential fuel to the body without controlling the need for so much insulin.

The Index

Foods are generally rated from 1 to 100. Those below 50 (this includes cheeses and proteins) tend not to require insulin. Those foods that score 50–70 should only be eaten occasionally. Those foods over 70 are best avoided.

The ratings are based on a food's fibre content, its absorption speed and what type of carbohydrate or sugar it is. This all sounds very healthy, but there are problems. The system ignores nutritional values. Some examples being:

Mars bar and raisins are both 60–69
White rice and brown rice are both 80–89
Parsnips are 97, yet potato chips are only 75

To add to the confusion, the various G/I listings that one sees are not standardized. Some authors claim that carrots are 49, others say 97. There is a 40–50 per cent variation in many foods across the various lists.

As a rough guide to carbohydrates, the G/I has a certain value, but our own common sense is perhaps the best guide to food selection.

The Insulin/Glucagon Connection

Up to 10 years ago, insulin was only mentioned in the context of deficiency and diabetes. The concept of too *much* insulin was rarely discussed or considered as a health problem.

Insulin has been termed the 'storage or fattening hormone', as its role is to convert and store nutrients for future use. Before humans developed agriculture, food storage and regular eating patterns, they were hunter-gatherers. Similar to the big cats in Africa and India today, this usually meant having a large meal every 3–4 days. The ability to store our own food was then a vital survival strategy. Insulin transfers dietary carbohydrates into *glycogen*, which is stored in the liver and muscles. A certain amount of glucose is used immediately by the muscles for the production of energy. Unfortunately the modern carbohydrate-rich diet provides far too much glucose for the sedentary 21st-century man and woman. Our bodies can only store a small amount of excessive glucose as glycogen. The remainder is stored as fat.

Too much circulating insulin (hyperinsulinism) can also suppress the release of another hormone, called *glucagon*. While insulin is released by the beta cells of the Islets of Langerhans in the pancreas, glucagon is produced by the alpha cells of the same islets.

The chief role of glucagon is to stimulate the conversion of glycogen into glucose in the liver. In other words, glycagon releases stored body fat, thus allowing the body to convert stores into energy.

Excess insulin blocks this vital glycogen activity, so that your fat reserves cannot be used as fuel.

Judy's Story

Consultation

Judy's excessive weight was not her only symptom. She was also tired and depressed, with a severe sugar and chocolate addiction.

At the time she came to see me she was 42 years old and weighed 202 lb (92 kg) – at 5 ft 6 in (168 cm) tall, this gave her a BMI of 33 (well into the obesity range). Her other symptoms included a tendency to feel shaky and irritable before each meal, which was relieved by eating. In her own words, she experienced a 'permanent hangover' every morning. She had endured many years of stress, as she had a child with disabilities and a rather unsupportive, selfish husband. Her father, who had died recently, had Type I (insulin-dependent) diabetes, and she had a younger sister with mild Type II diabetes.

Although low blood sugar and diabetes may appear to be at opposite ends of the spectrum, they belong to the same family of conditions and low blood sugar frequently precedes late onset diabetes. Many of my patients with low blood sugar have a parent, sibling or grandparent with diabetes.

Diet

Judy's diet was not good. With all her daily responsibilities, she had very little free time. She tended to cook convenience meals for her family. She also took very little exercise except housework. Her routine consisted of high sugar and refined carbohydrate foods, with 10–12 coffees each day with two teaspoons of sugar per cup. Judy ate chocolate every day, and consumed biscuits or cake on a daily basis. Her alcohol consumption (mainly dry sherry), was 4–6 units daily.

Diagnosis

I requested a series of blood tests including a thyroid profile, an anaemia check, blood fats and blood glucose levels. All the results were well within the normal ranges. I therefore requested a test that is rarely requested in the UK – a fasting blood insulin. Unless the patient attends the laboratory for the test, the serum needs to be posted in a special insulated box to maintain a low temperature. This is perhaps one reason why the test is rarely requested.

Test Results

Judy's result was very useful, as her insulin – at 41 mu/L – was twice the normal upper limit.

Judy's excess insulin was causing her body to store food as fat for later use. The only problem was she was not using her stored fat, now or later, and she was gaining weight. Insulin excess (hyperinsulinism) also tends to lower the blood sugar between meals, thus increasing the craving for sugar and chocolate. This explained Judy's shaky feelings before meals and why she felt so awful on rising.

Judy had followed many different diets over the previous few years without much success. The basis of these diets were usually low-fat, low-protein and high unrefined complex carbohydrates. This type of diet was totally inappropriate for Judy. A high-carbohydrate content actually stimulates the release of insulin. I can only assume that those who are successful on such a diet do not have hyperinsulinism, and do not have insulin resistance. All carbohydrates end up as sugar in the blood – only the speed of absorption, not the eventual outcome, is influenced by the type of carbohydrate we eat.

Treatment

I advised Judy to follow a low-carbohydrate diet (see page 48). The frequent drinks and late suppers would help her to stabilize her blood sugar.

I also prescribed two supplements for Judy, Carnitine 1,000 mg and the GTF Complex™ (see pages 51–52).

When I explained to Judy why she was so overweight and why she felt unwell at certain times, and why her previous diets had not worked for her, she gradually became more optimistic and enthusiastic. Her energy increased so that she felt able to swim three or four times each week.

Judy's weight loss was very gradual. Her use of sugar and fats as fuels needed to be converted to energy production instead of energy storage, and this can be a slow process. However, after four months her weight had fallen from 202 lb (92 kg) to 185 lb (84 kg), and at her last visit, which was nine months after her initial consultation, her weight was down to 162 lb (73 kg). This gave her a new BMI of 26, so that she was only borderline overweight.

Judy's case shows very clearly that there is no such thing as a weight-loss diet that works for everyone. It is sometimes necessary to choose a diet to address and remove the specific cause or causes of a person's overweight. This can be much more rewarding than simply eliminating fat and sugar or reducing the total calories.

Insulin Resistance

Many doctors and naturopaths who treat obesity, claim that insulin resistance is to be found in 70–75% of overweight people. Patients with late-onset or Type II diabetes (also known as non-insulin-dependent diabetes mellitus, or NIDDM) do not always suffer from insulin deficiency, but from a lack of sensitivity by their cells to insulin. This leads to the pancreas secreting more and more insulin in an attempt to control blood sugar levels successfully. When this occurs, and more insulin is produced, a vicious circle is soon established as the altered metabolism diverts calories into fat, particularly upper body fat. Unfortunately, as the weight increases, the insulin resistance also increases.

Syndrome X

This term has been used to describe a syndrome including insulin resistance, raised blood insulin (though blood glucose levels remain normal), high blood pressure, reduced HDL ('good') cholesterol and raised blood triglycerides (fats). Aside from blood measurements and other laboratory tests, those with Syndrome X usually show a raised waist to hip ratio, a raised BMI, oily skin and excess body hair. (Women with a diagnosis of PCOS (see Chapter 8) often have a parallel hyperinsulinism and syndrome X as well.)

Diabetes and Your Weight

Having described low blood sugar, raised blood insulin, insulin resistance and Syndrome X, and how all can lead to excess weight, it is perhaps tempting to assume that low blood insulin (diabetes) would cause weight *loss*. Unfortunately this is not so, as around 70% of people with diabetes are overweight.

So why are people with diabetes given drugs or actual insulin by injection to increase their insulin levels? Because many people with

Type II diabetes suffer insulin resistance, which means they need more and more insulin to maintain their blood sugar control.

There are two major variations of diabetes:

1   Type I (insulin-dependent diabetes mellitus, or IDDM). This group accounts for approximately 10% of all people with diabetes.
2   The larger group (90%) are people with Type II diabetes (also known as non-insulin dependent diabetes mellitus, or NIDDM). This is also sometimes termed 'late-' or 'maturity-onset' diabetes.

In Type I, a lack of insulin raises the blood glucose levels.

In Type II, a lack of insulin sensitivity raises the blood insulin *and* the blood glucose levels. Those in this group are usually over-weight, which can lead to further insulin resistance.

Diabetes and Health

Obesity is seen as the single main cause of Type II diabetes. Around 20% of the population is seriously overweight, and cases of diabetes are increasing every year. Overeating, especially of sugar-rich and high-fat foods, can lead to excessive demands on the body's sugar-regulating apparatus, and the pancreas can become exhausted and underactive. The modern tendency to refine foods, particularly carbohydrates, allows our appetite control to be by-passed. In primi-tive societies sugar was consumed occasionally as honey, but chiefly as a hidden ingredient of fruits, vegetables and grains. Eating such foods in their natural state ensured that too much sugar could not be consumed, as its input was naturally controlled by the appetite.

People with Type II diabetes tend to develop health problems that are normally associated with premature ageing. These include early blindness, kidney disease (with subsequent kidney failure), poor cir-culation, heart disease, and neurological disorders. Sometimes, even several years before a diagnosis is made, the poor control of glucose and insulin has an impact on health, resulting in female hormone disorders, blood pressure changes, loss of libido, fatigue and obesity. The poor circulation that accompanies diabetes can also contribute to muscle and joint pain and stiffness.

Glucose is the chief fuel for the body's cells. Although our brains account for around 3% of our body weight, the total consumption of available glucose by the brain is up to 20%. It is therefore not surprising that when our blood sugar control becomes faulty, learning, memory and mood can all be adversely influenced.

Insulin v Sugar

In Type II diabetes, the blood sugar rises because the cells have become resistant to the effects of insulin, and more and more insulin is released by the pancreas in an attempt to move the sugar from the blood and into the cells. It is the raised blood insulin that causes the high LDL ('bad') cholesterol, high triglycerides (blood fats), raised blood pressure, heart disease, poor circulation and obesity. However, late onset diabetes and hyperinsulinism can be improved with a strict low-carbohydrate diet (see pages 48–51), coupled with the support of specific nutritional supplements.

As a general rule, people with diabetes tend to convert food to fat instead of energy. Statistically, many health problems are more frequent or more severe if diabetes is present.

One sign of excess weight associated with diabetes is that it is often gained on the hips.

Waist-to-hip Measurement Ratio

Your waist-to-hip ratio should not be greater that 0.8. A greater ratio can predispose you to heart disease, osteoporosis, diabetes and osteoarthritis.

The measurement is calculated as follows:

Waist measurement (at narrowest) divided by hip measurement (at widest) – for example, 32 in (81 cm) waist divided by 38 in (96 cm) hip = 0.84.

When calories are stored as fat, blood pressure and cholesterol are usually raised. The food energy is stored and not available for daily use, so even a so called 'high-energy diet' does not always provide sufficient energy. When the 'switch' from energy use to energy storage occurs in this way, a normal calorie input can increase your weight, and weight-reduction diets just do not seem to be effective. The frustrated weight-watcher resorts to starvation diets, weight-loss remedies, overzealous exercise programmes or mono-diets in an effort to reduce the increasing weight.

Treatment Plan for Diabetes

Diet
People with diabetes need to restrict the sugar in their diet because they cannot produce sufficient insulin to maintain a normal, healthy blood sugar level, or because they are insulin-resistant. The following guidelines are useful for anyone with diabetes.

Protein	15–25% of your diet, which should consist mainly of plant proteins, fish and fowl (with the skin)
Carbohydrate	50–60%, consisting mainly of unrefined legumes, cereals, vegetables and fruit
Fat	20–25%, consisting chiefly of polyunsaturated fats, flaxseed oil and fish oil (omega 3)

The quality and choice of proteins, carbohydrates and fats should, however, take precedence over any rigid percentage-basis for diet planning.

Refined foods require a much higher insulin response when compared with unrefined foods. Plant proteins and fish produce a lower insulin response than fatty animal meats. Fibre-rich unrefined vegetables and cereals also reduce the insulin response.

Try to have plant proteins each day. Avoid concentrated fruit juice (always dilute with 50% water) and all sugar-rich foods.

Avoid convenience foods, fat-rich foods, fried foods and hydrogenated margarines. Cut all fat from your meat, and reduce your full-fat dairy foods.

Exercise
There is more about exercise in Chapter 11, but people with diabetes – and anyone with poor glucose-insulin control – need to exercise for 20–30 minutes each day.

Harry's Story

Consultation

Harry was a 68-year-old with adult onset Type II diabetes. Although he claimed to have 'stable' diabetes, he suffered from very poor circulation to his legs and feet. He also experienced frequent throat infections, and was tired and overweight. The fatigue had been with him for 2–3 years and he had been overweight for 8 years. He had been diagnosed with diabetes 12 years earlier, and he had been using insulin for 11 years.

His weight when he came to see me was 232 lb (105 kg), and he was 6 ft 2 in (188 cm) tall, giving him a BMI of 30 (just at the lower end of the 'obese' range). Perhaps not surprisingly, Harry's blood pressure was raised. In my book *Why Am I So Tired?*, which deals with mild hypothyroidism (underactive thyroid), I have written:

> *I find that low thyroid function is more frequently found in diabetics than in non-diabetics. It is also worth remembering that although insulin injections may provide adequate control of the blood sugar levels, it does nothing to reduce the secondary symptoms of diabetes.*

Significantly, many of the complications that develop as a result of diabetes also occur in hypothyroidism without diabetes. These symptoms can involve the nervous system, muscles, eyes, kidneys, joints and, perhaps most seriously, the heart and circulatory system and the weight.

Diagnosis

To understand just how Harry's diabetes was adversely affecting his metabolism, I requested my standard test-profile for diabetes, plus a thyroid profile. This included the following:

General haematology and biochemistry
Serum mineral profile
Essential fatty acid (blood) profile
Serum fasting insulin levels

Results

Harry's results showed the following abnormal readings:

Minerals	Low levels of magnesium, zinc and chromium
Essential Fatty Acids	Omega 6 (Linoleic Acid/LA) was deficient Omega 3 (Alpha Linolenic Acid/ALA and Eicosapentaenoic Acid/EPA) were deficient
Biochemistry	The total cholesterol and triglyceride levels were both raised, and the glucose level was above the normal reference range
Thyroid profile	Harry showed a border-line hypothyroidism
Insulin	Harry's fasting insulin was 20% above the normal upper limit. Together with his raised blood glucose, there was little doubt that Harry showed a tendency to insulin resistance.

Treatment

DIET

Harry's diet was not ideal for his present state of health. he considered that all carbohydrates were permitted if they were not refined. This meant that he ate brown rice, wholemeal bread and cereals, and wholegrain pasta on a regular basis. I advised him to reduce his carbohydrates to a minimum and to eat more fish and offal meats (to increase his intake of Omega 3 and 6, zinc and carnitine).

In addition, I advised he take the following supplements (see also pages 51–52):

Biotin
Thyro Complex™ (nutritional thyroid support; see Chapter 9)
Carnitine (fat-burner protein; see Chapter 6)
Vitamin E (to assist peripheral circulation)
Vitamin C (anti-oxidant)
Magnesium glycinate
Chromium polynicotinate
Zinc picolinate
Flax seed oil (freshly extracted from 3 tablespoons of seeds each day)

FLAX SEED OIL

Defined by Dr Robert Atkins as 'The king of vegetable oils' and by Udo Erasmus as 'a wonder grain of health', this valuable plant has been in use for 7,000 years. Flax seeds cannot be digested, being protected by a very thick seed coat. However, if you grind the whole flax seeds you obtain the best oil. You also obtain flax-seed meal, which contains many minerals, vitamins and lignans (valuable for treating bacterial, viral and fungal infections). The fresh oil of flax seed is the richest known source of Omega 3 essential fatty acids (EFAs). However, it becomes rancid (it is known as linseed oil) when exposed to light, heat or oxygen. Freshly extracted flax seed oil loses its fresh taste within 2–3 days if exposed to light and air.

Flax seed oil is prescribed for those with high blood triglycerides (fats), cancer, arthritis, diabetes, obesity, heart disease, PMS and many other health problems. Significantly, flax seed oil is known to reduce the insulin requirements of people with diabetes. The antioxidants Vitamin B_3, B_6 and Vitamin C and the minerals magnesium and zinc are essential to prevent deterioration of the oil.

An ideal daily dose would be 1–6 tablespoons of flax-seeds (taken with up to 5 times the seed's weight in water – 1 tablespoon of flax seed provides approximately 1 teaspoon of oil).

A mix of seeds and fresh bottled flax seed oil is usually advised if more than 4 tablespoons of ground seeds are recommended as a daily quota. As Udo Erasmus says in his book *Fats That Heal, Fats That Kill*, 'properly made fresh flax oil, or balanced blends containing it, ought to become part of the intake of virtually the entire population'.

FOLLOW-UP

Both Harry and I knew that his progress would be slow. We also knew that his metabolism needed to be more balanced and more efficient before any permanent weight reduction occurred. I requested another blood test to look at his blood fats, sugar and thyroid, four months after the initial consultation. There was already a general improvement. Harry himself was beginning to feel less tired and he had lost 18 lb (8 kg) in weight; being down to 214 lb (94 kg) – a BMI of 27.5 (still overweight but below the 'obese' range). Harry would never be slim, but we both hoped that he could lower his weight to achieve a BMI of less than 25. Such a weight loss would rebalance his sugar and fat metabolism, improve his blood chemistry and also lower his blood pressure.

Chapter Summary

1 Low blood sugar (hypoglycaemia) and high blood sugar (diabetes) can both result in excess weight.
2 Many systems in the body malfunction if the available sugar in the blood is too high or too low.
3 Tests are available to measure an individual's response to glucose. (However, single random blood sugar tests are of little value.)
4 Insulin resistance and Syndrome X play a major role in sugar metabolism.
5 Simply avoiding sugar is not the only treatment. Many specific nutrients play a part in sugar metabolism.
6 When your blood sugar is within the narrow band that is recognized as normal, there is every chance of your weight returning to normal.

Diets for Low Blood Sugar and Diabetes

Here I've set down a diet for those whose low blood sugar levels are contributing to weight gain – which can be used for meat-eaters, vegetarians or vegans – and a diet to be followed by those with diabetes or hyperinsulinism who need to stick to a low-carbohydrate diet.

Please note that the Lunch and Dinner options can be reversed if this is more convenient for you.

I have also included a list of valuable Dietary Supplements – see pages 51–52.

Diet for Low Blood Sugar

On Rising
    1 piece of fruit or 5 fl oz (1/4 pint/150 ml) fresh fruit juice

Breakfast
   1 piece of fruit or 4–5 fl oz fresh fruit juice
   Selection from the following:
   Egg (scrambled, poached, boiled or an omelette)
   Sugar-free baked beans, sugar-free ham or grilled bacon
   Cheese, sardines, mushrooms, tomatoes, vegan paté (Tartex) or
      vegan cheese on toast
   Grilled or steamed fish with one slice of wholemeal bread, or two
      Ryvitas with butter or soya margarine
   Wholegrain cereal or muesli with milk, soya milk or yoghourt
      and fresh fruit
   Natural yoghourt, milk or beverage (herbal tea, decaffeinated
      coffee, weak China or Indian tea) to drink

2 Hours after Breakfast
   5 fl oz fresh fruit juice (with protein drink or tablets if prescribed)

Lunch
   Meat, fish, (vegan) cheese, eggs, vegetarian/vegan savoury, rice,
      nuts or fruit
   Mixed fresh salad (large serving of lettuce, tomato, cucumbers,
      etc.) with French dressing, mayonnaise, cider vinegar, lemon-
      juice or sugar-free mayonnaise
   1 slice of wholemeal bread, toasted, or 1–2 Ryvitas with butter or
      soya margarine
   Dessert (optional) – cheese, yoghourt or fruit
   Beverage, as breakfast

2 Hours After Lunch
   5 fl oz fresh fruit juice, (with protein drink or tablets if
      prescribed)
   (and every 2 hours thereafter until Dinner)

Dinner

Home-made soup if desired

Mixed vegetables or salad

Liberal portion of meat, fish or poultry, or vegetarian/vegan
savoury, which can include a cheese or egg dish, stuffed
peppers, tomatoes, mushrooms, aubergines, courgettes, vegan
cheese dish, savoury rice, vegetable pie or casserole; lentil
savouries, soya dishes or wholegrain pasta

1 slice of wholemeal bread if desired

Dessert – cheese, yoghourt with Ryvita; stewed, baked or fresh fruit

Beverage, as breakfast

2 Hours after Dinner

5 fl oz fresh fruit juice, milk or soya milk or a small handful of
unsalted nuts (with protein drink or tablets if prescribed)
(and every 2 hours until Supper)

Supper

(as late as possible)

Protein snack is essential. Cheese, ham or cold meat, veggie/
vegan paté or cheese or soya milk with Ryvita or bread with
butter or soya margarine

Beverage or (soya) milk

Low Carbohydrate Diet

On Rising

1 piece of fruit or 5 fl oz (1/4 pint/150 ml) fresh fruit juice

Breakfast

1 piece of fruit or 5 fl oz fresh fruit juice

Selection from the following:

Egg (scrambled, poached, boiled or an omelette)

Sugar-free baked beans, sugar-free ham or grilled bacon

Cheese, sardines, mushrooms or tomatoes on toast

Grilled or steamed fish

1 small slice of wholemeal bread, or 2 Ryvitas with butter or soya margarine

Natural yoghourt, milk or beverage to drink

2 Hours after Breakfast

5 fl oz fresh fruit juice

Lunch

Meat, fish, cheese or eggs, salad (large serving of lettuce, tomato, etc.) with French dressing or mayonnaise, vegetables if desired. Only 1 small slice of wholemeal bread, toasted, or 2 Ryvitas with butter or soya margarine.

Dessert – Cheese, yoghourt or fruit

Beverage

2 Hours after Lunch

(and every 2 hours thereafter until Dinner)

5 fl oz fresh fruit juice

Dinner

Soup if desired, vegetables or salad, liberal portion of meat, fish or poultry, only 1 small slice of wholemeal bread if desired

Dessert – Cheese, yoghourt or fruit

Beverage

2 Hours after Dinner

(and every 2 hours until Supper)

5 fl oz of fresh fruit juice or milk or small handful of unsalted nuts

Supper
   (as late as possible)
   Ryvita with paté, cheese, ham or cold meat with butter or soya
      margarine
   Beverage or milk

Notes
If the dairy products are unacceptable due to catarrh or migraine, substitute soya milk, plant milk or other non-animal products.
   It is advisable to avoid the use of sugar substitutes.

Allowable Food and Drink

VEGETABLES
Asparagus, beets, broccoli, Brussels sprouts, lettuce, mushrooms, nuts, cabbage, avocados, cauliflower, carrots, celery, sweetcorn, cucumber, beans, onions, peas, radishes, sauerkraut, tomatoes, turnips, swede, parsnips and any other vegetables not on the AVOID list (see opposite).

FRUITS
Apples, apricots, bananas, berries, grapefruit, melons, oranges, peaches, pears, pineapple, tangerines and any other fruit not on the AVOID list. May be cooked or raw, but without sugar.

JUICES
Any unsweetened fruit or vegetable juice.

BEVERAGES
Any natural coffee substitute or decaffeinated coffee. Herbal teas or weak China or Indian tea.

DESSERTS

Fruit (fresh, stewed or baked). Yoghourt, cheese and sugar-free natural desserts.

ALCOHOLIC & SOFT DRINKS

Generally best avoided, but 'Slimline' sugar-free and dietetic drinks may be taken occasionally.

Alcohol should be limited to an occasional glass of dry white wine with the main meal.

Avoid

Any foods not mentioned on the diet and in particular sugar, chocolate and other sweets, etc., such as cakes, pies, pastries, sweet custards, puddings, ice cream, as well as salted nuts and all cereal products, syrup, molasses and honey.

Caffeine, ordinary coffee, strong tea, beverages containing caffeine.

Potatoes, grapes, raisins, plums, figs and dates.

Avoid tinned or bottled fruit juice unless sugar-free.

Tobacco.

Supplements

Carnitine

This fat-burning protein speeds fat oxidation and is a valuable adjunct for people on a weight-loss programme. The more Carnitine available to the body, the speedier fat is transported and oxidated into energy. It also assists in reversing the body's storage role for fat. (See also Chapter 6.)

GTF Complex™

This supplement was formulated by me several years ago for Nutri. The ingredients are all of value in treating low blood sugar. For readers' interest, here is a list of its ingredients:

Magnesium (citrate)
Thiamin HCI
Vitamin C (as ascorbic acid)
Manganese (aspartate)
Potassium (aspartate)
Riboflavin
Calcium (citrate)
PABA
Vitamin E (as d-alpha acetate)
Zinc (aspartate)
Pantothenic acid (as pantothenate)
Vitamin B_{12} (as cyanocobalamin)
Choline (bitartrate)
Vanadium (vanadyl sulphate)
Adrenal (freeze-dried) (Bovine)
Pituitary (anterior) (Bovine)
N-Acetyl-Cysteine
Chromium (nicotinate)
Niacin (as niacinamide)
Parotid (freeze-dried) (Bovine)
Inositol
Folacin (as Folic acid)
Vitamin B_6 (as pyridoxine HCL)
Biotin

CHAPTER THREE

Fats and Your Weight

Most of us, particularly if we are overweight, have an instinctive fear of fats. Fat consumption is of course often linked to obesity, heart disease, cancer and diabetes. We tend to regard fats as nutritionally useless and potentially dangerous. Yet in spite of the current fat-phobia and the popularity of low-fat diets, obesity in most Western nations is on the increase.

Any food or supplement supplier knows that the magic words 'fat-free' will boost sales of their product. The public assumption is that by avoiding fat, you will lose fat and lose weight. This is a false assumption, as there are good fats and bad fats.

Good Fats and Bad Fats

First, the facts:

1 Your metabolism can be increased and weight loss can be achieved by taking supplementary fats.
2 Essential fatty acids (EFAs) are, as a group, the chief nutritional deficiency in Western diets.

Some types of fat are essential to your health. In spite of a general reduction in the fat content of Western diets, conditions such as obesity, heart disease and diabetes are all on the increase. As fats are so important to your health and can provide useful supplements for many health problems – including excessive weight – it may be worthwhile taking a quick look at the fat family.

Saturated Fat	*Unsaturated Fat* Omega 6	*Mono-Unsaturated Fat* Omega 3
	Sources	
Meat	Linseed Oil	Fish (cold water)
	Safflower Oil	Flaxseed Oil
	Sunflower Oil	Rapeseed Oil (Canola)
	Corn Oil	Soyabean Oil
	Evening Primrose Oil	Walnut Oil
	Borage Oil (Starflower)	Wild Game
	Blackcurrant Seed Oil	
	Containing these EFAs	
	Gamma Linolenic Acid (GLA)	Alpha Linolenic Acid (ALA)
	Linoleic Acid (LA)	Eicosapentaenoic Acid (EPA)
		Docosa-Hexaenoic Acid (DHA)

Fats are all termed *lipids*. A fat is the type of lipid that is *solid* at normal room temperature. If a lipid is liquid at room temperature, it is called an *oil*.

Essential Fatty Acids

The word 'essential' in Essential Fatty Acids is used to describe a substance that the body cannot itself manufacture. EFAs must therefore be obtained from our food. They are necessary for human health and are grouped into several families, the Omega 3 and Omega 6 fats being the most important.

Saturated and Unsaturated Fatty Acids

You will have noticed that the Omega 3 and Omega 6 fatty acids are termed 'unsaturated' fats, while the animal fats are known as 'saturated'. What do these terms mean?

Saturated Fatty Acids

The chemistry of fats is a complex subject, and not essential or appropriate for a book on weight. Suffice to say that the saturated fats, are chiefly derived from animal products in our diet, including beef, lamb, pork, ham, bacon, cream, butter, cheese, sausages and yoghourt. These fats (also known as trans-fatty acids) are rigid, being solid at room temperature and difficult for our body to metabolize. They reduce our ability to metabolize the beneficial, unsaturated fats efficiently, and contribute to many health problems including heart and blood vessel disease, obesity, blood-clotting, stroke and diabetes. Excessive sugar in the diet, by the way, is converted into saturated fatty acids.

WHAT ABOUT MARGARINE?

Margarine is manufactured by a process known as hydrogenation. With this method, cheap, poor-quality oils are converted to solid, spreadable, unnatural fats with a longer shelf life.

Udo Erasmus, in his book *Fats That Heal, Fats That Kill*, states:

When we hydrogenate oil, to make margarines and shortening, we systematically and preferentially destroy the only essential nutrients left in the oil. Natural, healthy oil is converted into unsafe transfat. Unfortunately the very low production costs for margarine allow it to be cheaper in the shops than butter and the high profits result in intensive media advertising.

Saturated fatty acids interfere with the normal metabolism of the EFAs. They tend to elevate the total cholesterol and the levels of 'bad' cholesterol (known as low-density lipoprotein, or LDL) in the bloodstream, and to reduce the levels of 'good' cholesterol (high-density lipoprotein, or HDL) – see 'The Cholesterol Controversy' (page 57).

To return to Udo Erasmus, he concludes that:

Since trans-fatty acids have detrimental effects on our cardio-vascular system, immune system, reproductive system, energy metabolism, fat and essential fatty acid metabolism, liver function and cell membranes, we should consider margarines, shortenings, shortening oils and partially hydrogenated vegetable oils to be harmful to human health!

Symptoms of a Lack of EFAs

There are many deficiency symptoms that can develop from a lack of the EFAs known as LA (Linoleic Acid – Omega 6) and ALA (Alpha Linolenic Acid – Omega 3):

Linoleic Deficiency Symptoms	*Alpha Linolenic Deficiency Symptoms*
Joint and muscle pain	Fatigue
Poor blood flow	High blood pressure
Eczema	Raised blood fats

Hair loss
Poor immunity
Poor wound-healing

Infertility

Kidney and liver inefficiency
Disturbance in behaviour
Overweight

Fluid retention
Immune dysfunction
Paraesthesia in limbs (pins
and needles sensation)
Changes in learning and
behaviour (particularly in
children)
Poor co-ordination
Accelerated blood-clotting
Overweight

These deficiency symptoms serve to highlight the important role of the Omega groups in human health. A deficiency of these vital EFAs has a depressing effect on our metabolism. The symptoms also listed show a remarkable similarity to the symptoms of another common health problem, hypothyroidism (see Chapter 9).

Measuring EFAs

The blood measurement of the EFAs, including Omega 3, Omega 6, Omega 9 and other fatty acids, is now included in the laboratory guide of many laboratories. This means that with a single blood test most of the EFAs can be accurately measured. Although dietary assessment and analysis of a patient's eating habits can be useful indicators of EFA consumption, a blood test offers more definitive information. Furthermore, with a follow-up test after appropriate supplement use, progress can be confirmed.

The Cholesterol Controversy

We are frequently told that a high level of cholesterol in our blood is bad for our health. But there are good and bad cholesterols, just as there are good and bad fats for us.

We are also told that we can be deficient in cholesterol, and low levels have been linked to depression and suicide, autoimmune diseases, cancer, anaemia, immune inefficiency and hyperthyroidism (overactive thyroid).

Cholesterol is needed by the body to make the female hormones oestrogen and progesterone, and the male hormone testosterone. The adrenal hormones cortisone, cortisol, DHEA and pregnenolone, and the fluid-regulating hormone aldosterone, are also made from cholesterol.

Cholesterol's other uses in the body include vitamin A synthesis, and help with the digestion of the fat-soluble vitamins A, D & E. Our skin secretes cholesterol, playing a protective, lubricating and repairing role.

As with 'fat-free', the marketing description 'cholesterol-free' is a powerful and persuasive term used to boost sales of certain foods, oils and margarines. Many of us link cholesterol to heart disease, yet 97% of the population can control their own blood cholesterol by changing their diet.

It is worth remembering that, although cholesterol is essential to human health, only 10–20% of our total cholesterol is obtained from food – the remaining 80–90% is manufactured by our livers. The body manufactures around 1,500 mg of cholesterol each day, and virtually every cell in our body contains cholesterol. Hence the generally poor response to 'low-cholesterol' foods.

Levels of cholesterol in the bloodstream become elevated if we are one of the unfortunate 1% who from birth produce excessive amounts (a syndrome called *familiar hypercholesterolaemia*) or follow high-sugar and high-calorie diets. Also, cholesterol levels increase when we are stressed, for the simple reason that cholesterol is a component or precursor of the adrenal stress hormones.

Eliminating Cholesterol
Although our body can make cholesterol, it cannot unmake it or break it down into components. Cholesterol is eliminated via our

bowels (as bile acid and cholesterol molecules). This process is more efficient if we have fibre in our diets. Very low-fibre diets cause up to 94% of the cholesterol to be reabsorbed, with a subsequent increase in our blood cholesterol levels.

Conclusions

After years of research (often subsidized by margarine manufacturers), the link between cholesterol, fat consumption and heart disease has still to be proved. The amount of cholesterol contained in our diets has barely changed over the last century. Yet in 1900, heart disease accounted for 15% of all deaths, while in the year 2000 this figure was 35%. We eat less fat, yet the incidence of conditions such as diabetes, strokes, cancer and obesity have all dramatically increased.

Framingham Research Project
This famous study, designed to identify risk factors in heart disease, studied the residents of Framingham in Massachusetts over a 30-year period. The researchers were able to demonstrate strong links between high blood pressure and heart disease, smoking and heart disease, and diabetes, obesity and lack of exercise with heart disease. However, they were quite unable to prove any connection between heart disease and diet – as they focused on their subjects' egg, meat and fat consumption. (What a pity the study did not include sugar!)

Fats and Losing Weight

The key to using supplementary fats to help weight loss involves the role of the body's two distinctly different types of fat cells: white fat cells and brown fat cells.

White Fat
This type of fat functions chiefly as energy storage and insulation. It accounts for up to 90% of the total body fat and is located just under the skin, especially around the buttocks, abdomen and thighs.

Brown Fat
This fat is found deep in the body and around the spine and vital organs. It owes its colour to *mitochondria* (heat-energy-producers within cells). Unlike white fat, which functions as an energy-storage system, brown fat makes up an energy-using system. Brown fat converts calories to heat, providing an energy source from the excess fat that we eat.

Age and Fats

The distribution of brown and white cells is set and determined in our genes, but the ratio of brown fat to white fat changes with age. The brown cells reduce in number as we get older, while the white fat cells increase. This in part explains why many of us tend to gain weight as we age.

When we lose weight, we reduce both brown and white fat cells – but when we regain lost weight, it is very possible that we chiefly regain white cells.

Thermogenesis

When brown fat receives the appropriate brain signals, any excess calories that are consumed are speedily and efficiently converted to heat and energy. When the brown fat stores are not efficient or are insufficient, our calories are converted to white fat and increased weight.

The human body normally functions at an optimal mouth temperature of 37 °C (98.6 °F) or an underarm, morning temperature of 36.6 °C (98 °F) (see Chapter 2 on Hypothyroidism).

Thermogenesis means 'the production of heat by metabolic processes'. I have already described the value of measuring the morning temperatures as a diagnostic clue to mild hypothyroidism. Although the ideal average is, 36.5–36.7 °C (97.8–98.2 °F), I regularly see patients (usually overweight patients) with an average temperature below 35.3°C (95.5 °F).

Those who suffer from a mildly underactive thyroid are always chilly with cold hands and feet, shivering fits and hypersensitivity to cold. They usually dread the onset of winter experiencing a worsening of all their symptoms, both mental and physical, between September and April.

Research is being done in Scandinavia to link the SAD Syndrome (Seasonal Affective Disorder) to hypothyroidism. The two conditions present similar symptom-pictures, including depression, body coldness, mental lethargy, reduced libido and fatigue. Significantly, most SAD victims experience a craving for carbohydrates, sugar and caffeine and claim to feel better after eating such foods.

One explanation for such mood improvement, is the increased production of the hormone serotonin. After eating carbohydrates, serotonin from the pineal gland in the front of the brain is converted to melatonin which is a hormone prescribed for the SAD syndrome, jet lag and other problems. Many of the anti-depressant drugs in common use, influence the availability of serotonin (also known as a neurotransmitter). Another possible reason for the sugar-cravings and feeling of wellbeing after consuming sugar-rich foods, is the role of the blood sugar. With hypothyroidism, low blood sugar is a common symptom. It is possible that those with SAD syndrome also suffer the symptoms of mild hypothyroidism.

Temperature and Weight

The link between hypothyroidism and a low body temperature may be our inability to burn fat into energy. An inefficient thyroid output can reduce metabolic efficiency and energy conversion. Many health problems that depress our metabolism can also depress our body clock (the thyroid gland.

So how can we persuade our bodies to change from fat storage to fat burning? To put this very simply, many overweight people convert excess calories to fat instead of energy. The result of such an inefficient use of food can include fatigue, body coldness and probably the chief symptom, overweight.

Fat Burning/Fat Storage

When brown fat receives the appropriate brain signals, any excess calories that are consumed are speedily and efficiently converted to heat and energy. When the brown fat stores are not efficient or are insufficient, excess calories are converted to white fat and stored.

If your body converts excess calories to fat instead of energy, the result of such an inefficient use of food can include fatigue, body coldness and, of course, overweight.

So how can you persuade your body to change from fat storage to fat burning?

Treatment

Carnitine (The Fat Burner)

Research into carnitine in the 1940s led scientists to class it as a member of the B vitamin complex family, and named it vitamin Bt. A vitamin, by definition, is a substance essential to the body which cannot be produced by the body and must therefore be supplied through the diet. Carnitine is in fact produced by the body, and is therefore a 'nonvitamin nutrient', closely related to the amino acids (proteins).

In his excellent book *Carnitine – The Bt Phenomenon*, Brian Leibovitz poetically defined carnitine's fat-burning property as follows: 'Carnitine is the shuttle that carries fat into the body's furnaces to be burned.'

We shall be hearing a great deal more about the value of carnitine in the years ahead, chiefly as a result of its three main therapeutic roles:

1 to assist heat energy and function
2 to improve muscle efficiency and strength
3 its application in weight control.

The body's rate of fat-burning depends on the availability of carnitine to transport the fat. Only this valuable but little-researched protein has the ability to 'shuttle' fats.

Dr Robert Atkins (a great fan of carnitine) has written:

One reason Atkins Center doctors prescribe carnitine so frequently is that it seems, in our experience, to be the nutrient most likely to overcome that bane of many dieters' existence, metabolic resistance to weight loss. For fat to be used up as fuel, carnitine is essential.

No doubt at some time in the future medical science will develop an efficient technique to remove white fat cells and replace them with brown fat cells. Until this occurs, it would be advisable to look at nutritional methods to encourage a better use of fat.

Fighting Fat with Fat

It may seem like a paradox to use supplementary fat to reduce body fat, but weight loss can be achieved by taking fats such as prostaglandins.

Prostaglandins
Many overweight people have a good proportion of brown fat spread throughout their organs and spine. Their problem, however, is the

efficiency of the brown fat and its rate of activity. Brown fat efficiency depends on specific substances known as *prostaglandins* (PGs). These are powerful hormone-like chemicals which act to regulate activity in the cells of the body. There are over 30 different types of prostaglandins; they have a very short life and each has a unique function. They are also, significantly, made from essential fatty acids (EFAs). Aside from their role in stimulating the mitochondria in the brown fat to increase fat-burning and energy production, the prostaglandins have many other vital functions.

The prostaglandin family is classified in three groups, or series, as follows:

Series 1   These are made from the Omega 6 EFA family, starting with linoleic acid (LA) as the first biochemical link.

Series 2   These again come from Omega 6 EFAs with the initial EFA link being also (LA), but they have a slightly different chemical profile.

Series 3   These are made from the Omega 3 EFAs, with Alpha Linolenic Acid (ALA) as the starting point in the production line.

The Functions of Prostaglandins
To highlight the importance of the PGs to human health, it may be a useful guide to list the functions of perhaps the most famous of the group, Prostaglandin E1 (or PGE1):

1   PGE1 reduces stickiness and clotting in the blood. Blood clots are thus minimized, so the risk of heart conditions and strokes is reduced.
2   It reduces insulin resistance, assisting blood sugar control.
3   It acts as a natural anti-inflammatory, and is of particular value with arthritis and allied conditions.

4 It improves our immune efficiency.
5 It acts as a diuretic by removing sodium (salt) and excess fluid via the kidneys.
6 It works as a vaso-dilator (blood vessel relaxor) and improves circulation, high blood pressure problems, cramp, claudication (cramp caused by over-use) and angina.
7 It assists in the body's regulation of the mineral calcium.

PGE1 is a powerful, versatile and vital chemical of which, in common with the other PGs, we are going to hear much more about in the future.

Problems in Production
Unfortunately the production of PGs from the Omega 3 and Omega 6 EFAs does not always work efficiently. There are various factors that interfere with, or even stop completely, this vital production line. These include:

1 High sugar diets
2 Zinc and chromium deficiency
3 Poor immunity and frequent infections
4 Ageing
5 High saturated fat diets
6 Diabetes
7 Fried foods
8 Alcohol
9 Diets rich in trans fatty acids (margarine, etc.)
10 Cooking oils (usually processed)
11 High cholesterol diets, rich in eggs, dairy products and red meat

The efficient conversion from EFA to the prostaglandins can be altered or blocked by any or all of these dietary influences. The options for change are either to address the 11 factors above, or to take the Omega 3 and Omega 6 EFA as supplements, and thus short-circuit and streamline the PG production line.

In a perfect world, lifestyle and dietary changes would seem the best answers, but taking supplementary GLA (the 'parent' of the PGE1 family) – and thus bypassing any block in the biochemical production line – would be the second-choice alternative.

To 'kickstart' your fat metabolism to an energy-converting mode instead of a storage mode, you may need to take a supplementary oil. The question is, what is the best source of the required oil: evening primrose, borage (starflower) or blackcurrant seed?

Evening Primrose Oil (EPO)
The only real drawback to EPO use is that it is only an Omega 6 oil, with no Omega 3 component. Sometimes the enzyme-blockages discussed above involve both Omega 6 and 3. You will need to take a source of Omega 3 with the EPO, the obvious choices being fish oil or flax seed oil. (Taking supplementary Omega 3 oil is never a bad idea in any case, as it is generally deficient in the Western diet.)

Borage (Starflower) Oil
Similar to evening primrose oil, borage contains only Omega 6 oil and therefore also needs the addition of fish oil or flax seed oil to complete the job.

Blackcurrant Seed Oil
This oil contains both Omega 3 and Omega 6 oils. It would therefore be the ideal choice as a supplement to assist fat-burning and PGE1 production.

Other Supplements of Value
When our metabolism converts GLA to prostaglandin E1, several other nutrients including magnesium, zinc, vitamin C and vitamins B_2 and B_6 must be present – either in your diet or, where needed, as supplements.

Simon's Story

Consultation

Simon was aged 53 years when he consulted me. His chief symptom was persistent headaches, usually made worse by any form of stress, and overweight. With a height of 5 ft 10 in (178 cm) and of medium build, he should have weighed around 168 lb (76 kg). For more than 10 years his weight had stuck at over 200 lb (91 kg). This was in spite of his low-calorie vegetarian diet. For many years, Simon's blood had shown raised cholesterol and raised triglycerides levels, coupled with high blood pressure. His father had died of a heart condition, suffering high blood pressure and overweight for most of his adult life. Simon's brother had recently experienced a mild coronary attack, and also suffered with elevated blood pressure.

Treatment

A way had to be found to reduce Simon's blood fats and stored body fats. Unfortunately, although he enjoyed a low-fat, high-fibre and low-sugar diet, his diet lacked two very important nutrients that are involved in the successful metabolism of fat: the amino acid (protein) carnitine, and the Omega 3 natural fatty acids.

The word carnitine is derived from *carn*, the Latin for 'flesh', relating to the fact that carnitine was first found in meat and is almost entirely derived from muscle meats.

Vegetarians, vegans and those who avoid animal proteins may be low in carnitine. This particularly applies as the amino acids lysine and methionine, which are both necessary for the synthesis of carnitine, are also very low in such diets.

The conversion to carnitine is dependent on vitamin C being available. Significantly, when vitamin C is deficient, blood fat levels are usually high as a result of the accompanying carnitine deficiency. For this reason vitamin C is usually prescribed when carnitine is prescribed.

Our livers can synthesize carnitine, but to quote Robert Atkins: 'While it's quite true that our bodies make this amino acid, rarely do we have enough to keep us at our healthiest.'

OMEGA 3S

The Western diet is usually deficient in these vitally important essential fatty acids. The EFAs found in the Omega-3 fats and oils are as follows:

- alpha linolenic acid (ALA) – found in hemp seed oil, flax seed oil, canola oil, soya bean oil, pumpkin seed oil, walnut oil and dark green leafy vegetables
- eicosapentaenoic acid (EPA) and docosahexaenoic acid (DHA) – found in fish (including salmon, trout, sardines and mackerel), animal brain, eyeballs, testes and adrenal glands. Chinese water snake oil is the richest source of EPA and DHA.

Simon was not willing to change his diet to include fish or red meat. The only answer to his high blood fats, high blood pressure and overweight was a planned supplement programme. He needed to burn off his fat and reduce weight in order to reduce his blood pressure. I therefore prescribed the following supplement programme:

L. carnitine	500 mg twice daily
Lecithin	1,300 mg daily
Choline	100 mg daily
Inositol	100 mg daily
Vitamin B$_3$	60 mg daily
EPA	240 mg daily
DHA	160 mg daily
Vitamin C	4 gm daily
Lipase	330 mg daily

LECITHIN, CHOLINE AND INOSITOL
These three nutrients assist the liver's fat handling. They help to burn fats and generally improve fat metabolism. They are termed *lipotropics*.
Lipase is a fat-digesting enzyme.

Conclusion
After four months on the supplements, Simon had lost 18 lb (8 kg). His blood picture had changed as follows:

Lipid Profile	at consultation	4 months later
Total cholesterol	7.8	6.3
HDL ('good') cholesterol	0.680	0.9
LDL cholesterol	5.4	4.6
Triglycerides	3.2	2.5

Simon's metabolism did not respond very well to a simple low-carbohydrate diet. Fats had built up in his system, probably as a result of inherited genetic factors. Only a concerted anti-fat supplement programme lead to eventual weight loss and an improvement in health.

Chapter Summary

1 Dietary fats are not always bad news for the overweight. There are good fats and bad fats.
2 Very low-fat diets can be unhealthy.
3 Essential fatty acids (Omega 3 and 6), from fish, flax and olive sources, are preferable to saturated animal fats.
4 Brown fat uses energy, white fat stores energy. Carnitine is a natural 'fat-burner'.
5 Cholesterol is an essential substance for health.
6 When our fat metabolism works well, weight loss is achieved and many associated symptoms can improve, particularly fatigue.

CHAPTER FOUR

Fluid Retention and Your Weight

Water, Water Everywhere

Approximately 55–60% of your body weight is fluid, so if you weigh 10 stone, up to 6 stone could be water. Why so much? Because the water content of the body has several important roles:

1 Water loss from the body is considerable, being lost as sweat, through breathing, and via our stools and urine. This loss acts as a cooling system (sweat), to flush out waste products (through the kidneys and bladder), and to facilitate normal, comfortable bowel movement (stools).
2 A major role of water is to transport important water-soluble nutrients (such as vitamins, minerals, etc.) throughout the body.
3 Our blood consists mainly of water, which acts to transport the blood constituents through the body.
4 Water assists the body's temperature control. Under conditions of extreme heat we can sweat several pints of water each day.

5 Saliva and the digestive juices both have a high water content. Over 12 pints can be required to make these vital juices, the water being recycled and returned to our tissues.

Water is not simply transported via blood vessels and other tubes, it is contained within the cells themselves. It is also found outside the cells. Many factors can lead to a build up of this extra-cellular fluid, which is usually associated with increased permeability of the walls of the small blood vessels. When we suffer from fluid retention we may be literally waterlogged, with perhaps 60–70% of our total weight consisting of fluid. Unfortunately fluid retention can also be subtle and widespread, thus making it sometimes difficult to identify as the cause of your excess weight. This chapter explains the many causes of fluid retention, how to find out if you suffer from fluid retention, and how to help yourself treat it.

Symptoms

How Do You Know If You Suffer Fluid Retention?

Virtually all the different tissues of the body have the capacity to store inappropriate fluid without showing obvious signs (i.e. looking irregular or any different from normal). Extra weight or a changed body contour can be caused by excess fat or fluid retention, and it is not always easy to differentiate between the two causes.

Severe fluid retention is known as oedema. As excess fluid usually gravitates to the legs, a simple test for this is to press firmly on the front part of your lower leg, just above the ankle. If the depression remains, your body is holding quite a lot of extra water. Other tests and observations are included in the following questionnaire, to help you decide if fluid retention is at the root of your weight problem.

Too Much Fluid – Yes or No?

1   Try the finger dent test on the bone just above your ankle. Any depression should clear immediately the pressure is removed.
2   If you wear rings, do they seem to have become smaller?
3   Have you noticed that your weight can increase by 1–3 pounds from morning to the end of the day? Such sudden weight shifts can only be caused by fluid retention. Therefore, check your weight on rising and on retiring.
4   Do your shoes become a tighter fit throughout the day, and if you remove your shoes in the evening do you experience difficulty if you then have to put them on again? Only fluid retention can make limbs swell so quickly.
5   Do you find that low-calorie dieting and regular exercise simply do not work for you as ways of reducing your weight?
6   If you are a woman, do you suffer from breast tenderness or weight-gain in excess of 2 pounds before your period?
7   Do you suffer from raised blood pressure?
8   Do you have a noticeably 'puffy' face on waking, which normalizes within a short time?

If your answer to one or more of these questions is Yes, there is a likelihood that you are retaining too much fluid, which could well be contributing to your excess weight.

What Causes Fluid Retention?

There are many health problems that can cause fluid retention or oedema, including:

1   Heart failure and thrombosis (blood-clotting), varicose veins and varicose ulcers.

2 Liver disease (cirrhosis).

3 Kidney failure or disease.

4 Protein loss, as is suffered in the case of burns, chronic diarrhoea or protein malnutrition (e.g. Kwashiorkor).

5 Histamine release – an acute allergy to certain foods or local allergic reaction to insect bites and stings.

6 Local restrictive pressure on blood flow caused by tight bandages, garters, and overtight plaster casts, etc.

7 An underactive thyroid (hypothyroidism) can lead to fluid retention as a result of poor circulation and coldness.

8 Drug side-effects as in the case of steroids (cortisone, etc.).

9 Obstruction of the lymph system (as with certain cancers) – the lymph system is a vast complex of transparently thin tubes, valves, nodes, ducts and specialized organs (such as the tonsils, thymus and spleen) which helps to protect and maintain the fluid environment of the whole body by producing, transporting and filtering lymph fluid. Perspiration and muscle contractions help pump the lymph throughout the system. The system also conveys fats, proteins and other substances to the blood, working in conjunction with the capillaries of the veins to normalize fluid balance. The lymph also transports lymphocytes, which are specialized cells that support the body's immunity.

Many less severe health difficulties can cause fluid retention, including various vitamin deficiencies – for example of thiamin (vitamin B_1), causing beriberi with oedema, pyridoxine (vitamin B_6), causing fluid retention and mineral (potassium) loss as a result of stress or a high-salt diet – as well as protein deficiencies, salt retention or hormonal imbalances. Recent evidence suggests that prolonged airflights can lead to deep vein thrombosis (DVT) as a result of pressure changes adversely affecting the circulation to passengers' legs.

Chronic stress has also been known to cause potassium loss via the kidneys, mainly as a result of adrenal exhaustion. As potassium loss can go hand in hand with an increase in sodium (salt) levels in the body, fluid retention can also arise.

Head injuries can result in oedema within the skull. Such a fluid build-up has a very similar effect to a brain tumour. The skull cannot expand, so the increasing pressure can cause brain damage.

Mountain sickness involves a swelling of the hands and feet. Mountaineers, skiers and hikers can develop this type of fluid retention, caused in part by a disturbance to the potassium-sodium balance in the body, as the metabolism is stressed at high altitudes. This leads to an inappropriate water distribution between the tissues and blood.

Food intolerances or sensitivities can lead to inflammation of the capillaries, resulting in increased gut permeability or leaking, and tissue waterlogging (see Chapter 6).

In severe cases, pulmonary oedema (accumulation of fluid in the lungs), can develop to the point of becoming life-threatening.

Drugs and Fluid Retention

Many prescription (and some non-prescription) drugs are known to cause fluid retention and resulting weight gain. You may wonder why drugs with known adverse side-effects are sold in the first place. The explanation is simple: If the therapeutic value of a drug exceeds its side-effects, then priority is always given to the clinical (and commercial) value. This is why you can buy paracetamol at any chemist, yet it is known that with some susceptible individuals 12 tablets can cause irreversible and fatal liver damage.

The lists below cite the common drugs that can cause or worsen fluid retention. I have provided their generic name, brand name(s), what they are used to treat, and the manner in which they can affect fluid metabolism. The majority of these drugs are prescription only, and if you are taking any of them, do not alter your dose without your doctor's approval.

General Name	Brand Name(s)	Used for	Effects on Fluid metabolism
ACE Inhibitors	Capoten	High blood pressure	Oedema caused by an allergic reaction
	Co-Zidocapt	Heart failure	Kidney damage leading to fluid retention
	Caporzide		
	Vascace		
	Innovace		
	Innozide		
	Staril		
	Tanatril		
	Carace		
	Zestril		
	Perdix		
	Coversyl		
	Accupro		
	Accuretic		

	Tritace		
	Triapin		
	Gopten		
	Odrik		
Anti-Virals	Aciclovir	Viral infections e.g. shingles	Kidney Damage leading to fluid retention
	Zovirax		
	Famvir		
	Valtrex		
Anti-Fungals	Fungilin	Candidiasis, Fungal infections	Can be toxic to the kidneys causing fluid retention
	Fungizone		
	Abelcet		
	Ambisome		
	Amphocil		
	Diflucan		
	Ancotil		

Grisovin

Sporanox

Nizoral

Daktarin

Nystatin

Nystan

Lamisil

Beta-blockers	Propranolol	High blood pressure, Anxiety, Angina, Thyrotoxicosis, Migraine, Heart rhythm disorders	Possible adrenal effects on the heart, leading to fluid retention from kidney inefficiency
	Inderal		
	Inderetic		
	Inderex		
	Secadrex		
	Atenolol		
	Tenormin		
	Co-tenidone		

	Kalten		
	Betaloc		
	Lopresor		
	Sotalol		
	Visken		
Calcium Channel Blockers	Tildiem	High blood pressure, Angina, Reynaud's phenomenon	As for Beta-blockers
	Plendil		
	Prescal		
	Motens		
	Zanidip		
	Cardene		
	Adalat		
	Nimotop		
	Syscor		
	Vertab		

Central-acting Antihypertensive drugs	Catapres	High B.P. (hypertension), Migraine	Fluid retention as a result of sodium retention
	Dixarit		
	Methyldopa		
	Aldomet		
	Physiotens		
Cephalosporins (antibiotics)	Distaclor	Bacterial infections	May result in an allergic reaction with resulting fluid retention
	Baxan		
	Ceporex		
	Keflex		
	Kefzol		
	Suprax		
	Mefoxin		
	Orelox		
	Cefradine		

Kefadim

Zinnat

Cortico Steroids	Prednisolone	Joint inflammation and pain, Asthma, Polymyalgia, Adrenal exhaustion, Allergic disorders, Skin conditions	Fluid retention as a result of sodium retention, General weight gain

Betnelan

Betnesol

Calcort

Dexamethasone

Decadron

Hydrocortone

Medrone

Kenalog

Co-Trimoxazole (antibiotics)	Septrin	Bacterial infections, pneumonia, etc.	Liver and kidney disorders e.g. nephritis
Danazol	Danol	Menorrhagia (heavy periods), Endometriosis	Fluid retention and weight gain, possibly caused by insulin resistance
Insulin	Actrapid	Diabetes (IDDM)	Fluid retention resulting kidney disorders and sodium retention
	Humulin		
	Humulog		
	Monotard		
Loop Diuretics	Lasix	Oedema (fluid retention)	Can result in low blood potassium levels, kidney damage and eventual fluid retention
	Burinex		
	Torem		

NSAIDS (non-steroid anti-inflammatory drugs)	Brufen	Pain and inflammation, chiefly of joints and muscles	Angio-oedema, fluid retention, occasionally kidney failure
	Fenbid		
	Emflex		
	Rheumox		
	Celebrex		
	Keral		
	Diclofenac		
	Voltarol		
	Diclomax		
	Arthrotec		
	Dolobid		
	Lodine		
	Lederfen		
	Fenopron		
	Froben		
	Indometacin		

Orudis

Mobic

Naprosyn

Synflex

Butacote

Feldene

Ponstan

Oestrogen	Premique	HRT	PMS-type fluid retention, Weight changes
	Premarin		
	Prempack		
Oestrogen & Progesterone (Low, standard & high strengths)	Many brand names	Oral contraceptives	Weight gain, fluid retention, other effects

Phenothiazines, Anquil etc.		Major tranquillizers used for schizophrenia, mania, brain damage, depression, delirium, anxiety, etc.	General weight gain, reduces heart & kidney efficiency leading to fluid retention
	Largactil		
	Depixol		
	Serenace		
	Promazine		
	Stelazine		
	Clopixol		
Potassium-sparing diuretics	Amiloride	Oedema (fluid retention)	Eventual worsening of fluid retention
	Dytac		

Progesterones and progestogens	Duphaston	PMS, Menorrhagia (heavy periods), Endometriosis, Contraceptive, HRT, Infertility	Can cause fluid retention as a result of sodium retention, insomnia, depression, alopecia, acne, period pain, PMS
	Proluton Depot		
	Provera		
	Utovlan		
	Primolut		
	Cyclogest		
	Gestone		
	Crinone		
Diuretics	Navidrex	Oedema (fluid retention)	Can lead to kidney disorders and fluid retention
	Hygroton		
	Hydrosaluric		
	Natrilix		

	Nephril		
	Diurexan		
Tricyclic anti-depressants	Amitriptyline	Depression	Can cause urinary retention. Allergic response may lead to fluid retention
	Lentizol		
	Asendis		
	Anafranil		
	Prothiaden		
	Sinequan		
	Tofranil		
	Lofepramine		
	Motival		
	Surmontil		
Vasodilators	Eudemine	High blood pressure	Can cause sodium and fluid retention
	Hydralazine		
	Apresoline		
	Loniten		

You may have thought that the side-effects of any prescription drugs you might be taking could constitute only a trivial percentage of your total excess weight. However, I have known patients to lose 15–20 pounds as a direct result of reducing, stopping or replacing their drugs. As I've said, however, you must always consult with your doctor before making any change to your medication regime.

Marion's Story

Consultation

Marion's chief reason for consulting me was her self-admitted 'obesity'. She was 30 years old and had put on 60 lb (27 kg) over the previous four years. She weighed 210 lb (95 kg) and was only 5 ft 2 in (158 cm) tall. This gave her a BMI of 39. An ideal weight for her height would be around 126–134 lb (57–60 kg).

Marion's other symptoms included period pain, with a reduced cycle of 25 days which included an 8–9 day bleed. Depression, fatigue and PMS completed her story.

Marion followed a high-fibre, low-sugar and low-fat diet. Recent blood tests had revealed a normal thyroid function. Her blood sugar, her kidney and liver tests all were within the normal ranges. Surprisingly Marion was not anaemic, in spite of her protracted bleed each month.

Marion was also taking two prescription drugs, both of which she had begun to take five years earlier. These were amitriptyline for depression and a progestogen, Norethisterone, which was prescribed for her irregular, painful periods. Unfortunately, a common side-effect of both drugs is fluid retention and weight increase.

While Marion felt that the anti-depressant was alleviating her depression, the Norethisterone did not appear to have much impact on her period symptoms.

I made contact with her doctor, who agreed with me that Marion's excess weight had itself became a causative factor for her various problems. He therefore agreed to discontinue her Norethisterone and to slowly wean Marion off the anti-depressant, with the understanding that I could begin to control her symptoms with plant remedies when she had stopped the amitriptyline.

Please note: It is never wise to stop medical anti-depressants abruptly, otherwise unpleasant withdrawal symptoms may develop. Always consult with your doctor first.

Although a great deal has been written about the benefit of St John's Wort to treat depression, I have found that a Kava Kava/St John's Wort combination is more effective and speedier in relieving the symptoms of depression, anxiety and insomnia.

I advised Marion to follow my low-carbohydrate diet and, in addition to taking Kava Kava and St John's Wort, I prescribed a course of plant-based (wild yam) progesterone cream that also contained the herbal remedies agnus castus, black cohosh, damiana and dong quai root. I have found this combination of plant remedies to be of great value when treating female hormonal imbalances.

Conclusion

It was two to three months before Marion was taking the full programme of plant remedies, and another three months before she began to feel less depressed and more healthy. Nine months after our first consultation she had reduced her weight to 171 lb (77 kg), with a BMI of 31 – still in the 'obese' range but certainly better than her original BMI of 39.

A full year after first seeing Marion, her weight was down to 147 lb (66 kg) with a BMI of 27. Her monthly symptoms were around 80% improved. Her moods were more stable, with only a slight pre-period irritability remaining.

Although drug side-effects can sometimes be blamed for weight gain, I find that other factors are also usually involved. Having said that, discontinuing or replacing the drugs is often a good first step to begin weight reduction.

Pam's Story

Consultation

Pam was a 32-year-old mother of two with three problems that concerned her:

1 She was overweight. At 5 ft 3 in (160 cm) tall, she weighed 181 lb (82 kg) – giving a BMI of 32 (well into the 'obese' range). She had been overweight since her first pregnancy, but only by about 7–10 lb (3–4 1/2 kg). In the previous 12 months, however, she had gained over 28 lb (13 kg).

2 Pam's blood pressure was too high. This had been diagnosed a year before; unfortunately her medication was not reducing the pressure.

3 Over the previous 9–10 months Pam had noticed that her ankles were swollen by lunchtime each day.

Pam's general health and vitality were good, although she admitted to becoming stressed easily with her two young children (aged 4 and 6).

I was curious to know why Pam's weight had ballooned so quickly the year before. Her swollen ankles suggested that she was retaining fluid, however she had no history of food sensitivities or intolerances, and her periods and bladder and kidney functioning all seemed quite normal. Upon checking, her diet was balanced, with no major faults (no excessive salt intake or low-protein regimes). Although she was eating only around 1,800 calories a day, she had failed to lose weight. The reason for her apparent fluid retention, overweight and high blood pressure remained a mystery until we began to discuss her medications.

A little over one year earlier, Pam's doctor had prescribed Atenolol, a beta-blocker, for Pam's raised blood pressure. The beta-blockers' action is not fully understood, but they are nevertheless prescribed for a large range of problems including migraine, high blood pressure, angina and heart rhythm disorders. They can adversely influence peripheral circulation to the limbs, and may cause fatigue. They also can reduce the heart's efficiency as a pump, which may compromise the kidneys' efficiency. It is this last side-effect that leads to fluid retention and weight gain.

Treatment

Pam's raised blood pressure, perhaps initially a product of stress, was now being made worse with her excessive weight. In the absence of any other obvious reasons for her sudden weight increase one year earlier, it seemed very possible that the Atenolol was the culprit. The weight increase coincided with the onset of the drug use.

I advised Pam to discuss her weight and fluid retention more fully with her doctor. He agreed to stop her beta-blocker for a short trial period, on condition that she lost weight. I prescribed an anti-stress formula that contained the plant remedies valerian, skullcap, passion flower and chamomile, coupled with adrenal tissue concentrate and the B vitamins. I also advised her to take a natural diuretic three times a day, to assist fluid loss. This is produced by Nutri Ltd and is a combination of vitamin B_6, potassium, kidney concentrate and the plant remedies dandelion, alfalfa leaf, fennel seed, shave grass, celery leaf and seed, and uva ursi leaf.

Conclusion

Pam's chief cause of her overweight was fluid retention, so her weight loss was speedy and dramatic. Within four weeks she had lost 16 lb (7.25 kg). When she returned for a progress report three months after our first meeting, her weight was down to 150 lb (68 kg) – a loss of 30 lb (13 kg) – and her BMI was just under 27. Her blood pressure had also fallen, and she said she felt more relaxed. Her doctor agreed to extend her avoidance of Atenolol. Pam had plans to join a gym, so I had no doubt that she would eventually reach her pre-motherhood weight of less than 140 lb (63 kg).

Not all patients retain fluid and increase their weight when taking prescription drugs. However, some individuals do tend to develop side-effects, among which fluid retention is not uncommon. Just another reason to explain stubborn weight loss.

Protein Deficiency and Fluid Retention

Protein deficiency can lead to fluid retention. This occurs when the protein called albumin is deficient in our blood. Albumin, which is produced by the liver from protein components, facilitates the passage of tissue fluid into the small blood vessels. In the absence of albumin, this fluid tends to stay in the tissues.

Significantly, serum albumin (blood albumin) also serves as a transport protein for the essential fatty acids, many drugs, and hormones including cortisol and thyroxine.

Amino Acids

The amino acids have been called the 'primary building blocks of life'. They are the chief constituents of protein (although some important amino acids are non-proteins). There exist over 100 amino acids, and new ones are still being discovered.

There are eight essential amino acids for adults, so-called because our body cannot make them and we must obtain them through our diet. They are: isoleucine, leucine, lysine, methionine, phenylalanine, threonine, tryptophan, and valine. Two other amino acids, arginine and histidine, are required in the diet of children and the elderly. The non-essential amino acids can be made by the body.

Proteins are essential to life and the body's continuous repair work, and replenishment depends on available amino acids. Our skin is replaced every 24–25 days. Most of the lining of the gastrointestinal tract (from mouth to rectum) is replaced every four days. Two and a half million red cells are made by our bone marrow every second. The majority of our white blood cells are replaced every 10 days. None of these processes can function without amino acids. Without the essential amino acids, we would begin to die.

The role of the proteins is well demonstrated by the heart-rending images of famine victims appearing on our television screens, showing children with Kwashiorkor (protein calorie malnutrition). These children have spindly limbs and muscle wasting with grossly enlarged stomachs, mental retardation and delayed growth. All these symptoms bear witness to the vital importance of protein in our diets.

Protein is in many foods, including meat, fowl, fish, milk, cheese, yoghourt, eggs, pulses (beans and lentils), and soya. Rice and cereals also contain protein. With so many sources, you may wonder just how you could possibly be protein-deficient. Here's how:

1 Following a vegan diet – particularly if you do not take advantage of the variety of plant proteins available
2 Fasting
3 Following a low-protein, all-fruit or raw foods diet
4 Being anorexic.

Nutritional deficiencies in human health are viewed by most of us as well defined, easily diagnosed and easily treated problems which (aside from iron-deficient anaemia) are usually seen only in third-world countries. They are often thought to be caused by wars, famine, plagues and other major catastrophes.

The true picture is very different, and a few statistics will show you just how much so. Government surveys in the US have shown that over 60% of the American population is deficient in one or more vital nutrients. In 1988 it was estimated in the American Surgeon General's Report on Nutrition and Health that 65–70% of all deaths in the US involved nutritional deficiencies.

It is not safe to assume that the affluent, industrialized Western nations all have non-deficient, varied or even appropriate diets for maintaining health.

American government surveys have shown that the only essential nutrient (of the 13 measured) present in adequate amounts was sodium. (Possibly resulting from the high salt content of many foods.) The Recommended Daily Allowance (RDA) defines the amount of a nutrient needed to avoid deficiency symptoms. Those who obtained less than the RDA essential vitamins and minerals are shown in the following table. (Clinical estimates of other nutrients are also included.):

Minerals	% less than the RDA	Vitamins	% less than the RDA
Calcium	68	A	50
Iron	57	B_1	45
Magnesium	75	B_2	34
Phosphorous	27	B_3	3
Chromium	90	B_5	25
Copper	85	B_6	80
Manganese	25	B_{12}	34
Selenium	55	C	41
Zinc	40–60	D	10
		E	30
		K	15

(Omega 3 deficiency – 95% estimated below RDA)

In 1956, a biochemist named Roger Williams wrote a book entitled *Biochemical Individuality* in which he stated that each of us is an individual, and unique, possessing a distinctive chemical composition. He showed that many of us function best when hormones, minerals, enzymes, proteins and vitamins are present in our bodies in above-average amounts and can be revealed in test readings to be at the upper end of the 'normal' range. This view leads to the obvious and easily provable conclusion that many of us suffer symptoms of nutritional or biochemical deficiency, even when our blood levels show us to be within the 'normal' range. While it is clinically and diagnostically useful to rely on normal ranges in order to identify the 'abnormal', after Williams' book the true nature of human diversity became obvious.

As I have already outlined, protein deficiency can lead to fluid retention and overweight. However, many other nutrients are involved in fluid control, including the Essential Fatty Acids, vitamins and minerals.

Treating Fluid Retention

As I have already outlined, protein deficiency can lead to fluid retention and overweight. However, many other nutrients are involved in fluid control, including the essential fatty acids (Chapter 3), vitamins and minerals. You must try to ensure that your diet is sufficient in all these vital nutrients.

How Much Fluid Do You Need?

The best treatment for combating fluid retention is to make sure you drink plenty of water. If you don't drink enough, the body holds on to what you do drink, instead of eliminating it. On average you should drink around 2 litres (3 pints) of water a day. Water acts as an appetite-suppressant and helps the body to metabolize stored fat. Those who are overweight need to drink more water. Cold mineral water is the preferred choice.

Chapter Summary

1 We all consist of 55–60% water, and can retain up to 70% or more tissue water. Many overweight individuals suffer with fluid retention from a variety of causes.

2 Water has many uses in the body, including nutrient transport, blood flow and temperature control. The important lymph system assists water re-cycling.

3 Successful treatment of fluid retention can only result from correct diagnosis of the causes. Taking drugs to reduce excess fluid and lose weight is only a temporary solution.

4 Overweight as a result of water retention may be a by-product of some other health problem such as an underactive thyroid (hypothyroidism, see Chapter 9), PMS, a high-sodium and low-potassium diet and/or a low-protein diet.

5 When our body's water percentage is normalized, weight loss is achieved. Unfortunately, although this type of weight loss can be achieved quite rapidly, without taking a good look at your general diet, you could put the weight on back just as fast.

CHAPTER FIVE

Candida Overgrowth and Your Weight

A tiny yeast parasite called *Candida albicans* is yet another common cause of excess weight. Although it inhabits the intestines of all of us, it is quite harmless – unless it proliferates for some reason and overgrowth (*candidiasis*) occurs. Although found mainly in the gastro-intestinal tract, which includes all tissues of the tract from the mouth to the anus, a candida overgrowth can invade other sites including the skin, the vagina and associated area, probably as a result of the proximity of the vagina to the anus.

Symptoms

The scope of candida's influence is complex and profound, so an overview of some of the symptoms and body systems affected may be of value.

Thrush
Visible candida, usually seen in the mouth, is termed 'thrush'. There is a tendency also to define vaginal candida as thrush. Thrush forms

a creamy-white, raised area consisting of a crumbly material not unlike milk curds or cream cheese.

Digestive Problems
Heartburn, Irritable Bowel Syndrome (IBS), stomach discomfort, diarrhoea or constipation and mucus or blood in the stools can be signs of candidiasis. Abdominal distention, rectal itching and – if the constipation is chronic – haemorrhoids can develop.

Women and Candida
Vaginal irritation and thrush, PMS with fluid retention and weight gain, loss of libido, bladder infections and endometriosis are all common symptoms – and effects – of candida in women.

Nervous System Problems
Poor memory and concentration are typical, often with general fatigue. Your sense of smell and taste may be altered. Poor hearing with tinnitus and vertigo, poor night vision and general clumsiness and reduced balance are also not uncommon.

Skin and Muscle Symptoms
Fungal infections of the skin, and skin and nail rashes may occur, particularly of the feet (e.g. athletes foot). Rheumatoid arthritis-type symptoms are also common in the presence of candidiasis, with stiff and painful joints and muscles, and muscular cramps and weakness.

Allergies
Food and environmental intolerances are fairly common with candidiasis. Tobacco smoke, perfumes, hair spray and many other sprays can cause symptoms. These usually disappear when the candida overgrowth is brought back under control.

Many symptoms of food intolerance can develop, including rhinitis, coughing, asthma, constant sneezing and post-nasal drip. Sore throats and repeated chest infections are quite common, as the immune system is weakened by the systemic candidiasis. Skin rashes, urticaria (hives), eczema and swelling of the lips and ears may occur (angio-neurotic oedema). Excessive reaction to insect bites, and skin irritations by contact with certain plants are also common.

(For more about Allergies and your weight, see Chapter 6.)

General Symptoms
This is a long list, but the following symptoms are all thought to be caused or contributed to by candidiasis:

- irritability and anxiety
- headaches
- depression
- bad body odour
- bad breath
- laryngitis
- bladder frequency (having to use the loo often) with burning
- insomnia
- body coldness
- low blood pressure
- excessive thirst
- pruritus (itching skin)
- night sweats
- ear infections
- low blood sugar symptoms
- swollen ankles at end of day
- numbness in fingers
- shortness of breath
- noisy stomach
- poor wound-healing
- underactive thyroid (hypothyroidism).

Readers will find that many of these symptoms are similar to the symptom-picture for an underactive thyroid (hypothyroidism – see Chapter 9). I find that candidiasis and hypothyroidism frequently co-exist, and a stubborn, vicious circle is often established that can be difficult to diagnose accurately and treat. A mutual aggravation is established between the two conditions, and simply treating either the thyroid *or* the candida is not very rewarding. It becomes essential to treat both disorders simultaneously to achieve the maximum benefit.

Gerry's Story

Consultation

When Geraldine, or Gerry as she preferred to be called, first consulted me she weighed 207 lb (93 kg). At 5 ft 5 in (165 cm), this gave her a BMI of 34 – well into the 'obese' range. She was aged 58 years and, in addition to being very overweight, she suffered from fatigue, depression, chronic indigestion and muscle stiffness and pain. She had been taking Hormone Replacement Therapy (HRT) for 12 years, and 50 mcg of thyroxine for a mild hypothyroidism for the previous 8 years. Unfortunately, Gerry also had Type I, late onset diabetes, and had been insulin-dependent for 2 years.

Gerry admitted to regularly 'forgetting' to have her insulin injection (which she should have had 4 times daily). She detested having to inject herself, so I thought it possible that this 'forgetting' was simply an excuse so she wouldn't have to do it so often. The result of this was a blood sugar level that at times was well out of control.

Gerry's blood pressure was 185/95, and her doctor had recently prescribed a hypertensive drug and the anti-depressant Prozac.

Tests

Recent blood tests had shown that her thyroid function was being controlled well, but that her cholesterol and triglyceride levels were much too high. A gut fermentation profile had shown an elevated ethanol (alcohol) level, double the normal range. This would be consistent with a yeast overgrowth.

Diet

Gerry admitted to a craving for bread and potatoes. In spite of this, her diet was quite well balanced in most areas. She had rather 'lost faith' in supplements and was, upon our initial meeting, taking only a yeast-free multi-vitamin-mineral capsule each day. She did not drink alcohol or coffee, did not smoke and, with her diabetes, she wisely avoided sugar and chocolates.

Diagnosis

Gerry was clearly suffering from candidiasis. Unfortunately her symptoms had been attributed to her hypothyroidism and diabetes. There was little doubt in my mind that her sugar-rich blood was a welcome source of food to a flourishing candida overgrowth. This initial diagnosis was then confirmed by her positive gut fermentation test.

Treatment

The priority was to stabilize Gerry's high blood sugar levels. I therefore stressed the importance of her sticking to her insulin regime. I advised her to check her glucose before each meal for the next 2–3 weeks, and then to set her insulin dosage and the carbohydrate level of the meal accordingly. This provided Gerry with a feeling of control over her diabetes, which she had been lacking. In a very short time her blood sugar levels were brought under control.

The next step was to discuss her HRT requirements with her doctor. Supplementary oestrogen is seen as a causative factor with candida overgrowth, whether the source of the oestrogen is HRT or the Pill. Her doctor was agreeable to a six-month trial period without HRT.

With the two chief causes of Gerry's candidiasis removed I could now concentrate on treating the actual problem. I prescribed the Exspore™ formula and discussed a few dietary changes. In many areas a diabetes diet and the anti-candidiasis diet are similar. I therefore advised Gerry to avoid yeast- and fungus-containing foods. I also advised her to begin simple daily exercises (initially cycling or swimming). I stressed the importance of not overdoing the exercises and further reducing her limited energy reserve.

Within 10 weeks Gerry's weight had fallen to 185 lb (84 kg), giving her a BMI of 30 – out of the 'obese' range. With her increased awareness of insulin dosages and blood sugar balance, her body was beginning to convert the sugar surplus to energy, and Gerry was beginning to pull out of her mental and physical depression.

After six months on the diet and supplements, Gerry weighed 160 lb (72 kg) – BMI 26. Her blood pressure readings were almost normal at 150/85, and she found she no longer needed to take the anti-depressant, Prozac.

Candidiasis: The Causes

We are host to six species of candida, of which Candida albicans is the most common. Beneficial bacteria – usually referred to as *acidophilus* bacteria – co-exist with and feed off the candida. When the friendly acidophilus control the candida, a balance is achieved. However, if the acidophilus are reduced or destroyed (as can be caused by taking antibiotics), or your immune system is suppressed or weakened (as with certain drugs and hormones), the candida proliferate to the level where symptoms begin to show.

Antibiotics

Modern broad-spectrum antibiotics are not specific – that is, they kill *all* bacteria, good and bad. The after-effects of such therapy can often be candidiasis. In many European countries (except Britain) this problem is recognized, and acidophilus capsules are prescribed along with antibiotics in an attempt to reduce the risk of candida overgrowth.

Unfortunately, over the last 40 years we as a society have all ingested a 'steady drip' of antibiotics (and low-dosage hormones) in commercially-reared poultry, pigs and beef. Antibiotics are routinely added to animal feeds. At one time traces were also detected in milk supplies, as a result of the frequent use of antibiotics to treat mastitis in cows.

Diabetes

People with diabetes are far more prone to candidiasis than those who do not have the disease. Bacteria (particularly candida) love sugar, so they see the sugar-rich person with diabetes' blood as a perfect fuel. The modern high-sugar diet is also a contributing factor. It is worth remembering that all carbohydrate foods end up as sugar in the blood.

Hormones

It is well known that some women only develop candidiasis when they are pregnant. Whether a result of immune suppression or hormonal fluctuations with pregnancy, the exact cause or causes are not known. Steroid use (e.g. cortisone) and the Pill have also been blamed for candida overgrowth. Any source of oestrogen (such as HRT and the 'morning-after pill') can also increase candida.

Other Causes

Other factors that can lead to an overgrowth of candida include stress, poor nutrition and inherited health factors, malabsorption, leaky gut syndrome – and virtually anything that depresses the efficiency of our immune system.

Stress

Stress of any kind, whether chemical, physical or emotional, can compromise our immune function. Adrenal efficiency, general vitality and the levels of the many nutrients that we require for health can be adversely influenced by stress. Prolonged stress can lead to immune system failure and subsequent candidiasis.

Poor Nutrition

Unfortunately, many of those who are anxious, stressed and fatigued tend to resort to comfort eating and drinking. This usually involves starchy snacks, coffee, alcohol and chocolate. So often in the early stages of many health problems, a vicious circle is established. Candida overgrowth often develops according to the pattern outlined here:

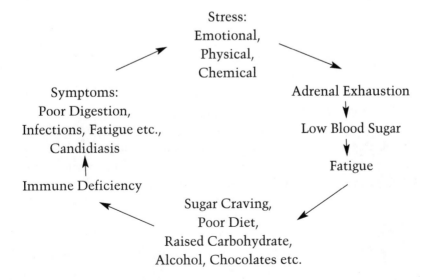

In my experience, candidiasis does not usually exist in isolation, but tends to develop as a component of a general 'syndrome' (*syndrome* being defined as a complex of signs and symptoms resulting from a common cause). The 'common cause' with candidiasis is a general lowering of vitality, immune efficiency and stress-handling.

Leaky Gut Syndrome
Although I will discuss this condition further in Chapter 6, it has a relevance to candidiasis. Candida overgrowth is seen as a common cause of leaky gut, along with parasitic infections, gut dysbiosis (intestinal bacteria imbalance), and drug side-effects.

Although essentially a simple yeast, when a candida overgrowth occurs and proliferates, the simple yeast develops into a fungal form. The fungal form has root-like structures known as *rhizoids*. This means that the candida changes from a relatively harmless and mobile simple yeast to a fungal form which literally 'takes root' in the intestinal mucosa or lining. Once the intestinal barrier is so breached (leaky gut syndrome), undigested food molecules (chiefly protein) can enter the bloodstream. These may not be recognized by our metabolism as food, triggering an immune defensive response in various tissues. When this occurs, the early stages of food intolerances may also develop.

Another end-result of candidiasis caused by a change in gut permeability is a tendency for bacteria, antigens (substances, usually proteins, that stimulate antibody production by the immune system, leading hopefully to immunity to the substance) and other harmful compounds to pass into the bloodstream. This can lead to local or systemic (whole-body) allergic responses. Bowel disorders, rheumatoid arthritis, food intolerances, liver toxicity and a wide range of conditions have been linked to the leaky gut syndrome, one of the chief causes of which can be candida overgrowth.

How Is Candidiasis Diagnosed?

Accurate diagnosis is not easy, because we all host a candida population within our intestines. Our immune systems will apparently tolerate a certain level of candida without symptoms arising.

The following questionnaire may serve to help you identify whether you have a candida overgrowth. Many practitioners who treat systemic candidiasis rely entirely on the patient's symptom-picture and history to diagnose the problem and assess its severity, the diagnosis being confirmed when symptom-relief is achieved. However, there are tests available to identify candidiasis and – perhaps of greater value – to assess the severity of the overgrowth. I shall discuss the relative value of these tests later in this chapter.

Candida Questionnaire

Part 1 – Possible Causes

ORAL CONTRACEPTIVES
Have you taken the birth pill for excess of 12 months within the last 2 years?
>   Yes/10 points
>   No/0 points

ANTIBIOTICS
Do you take them very occasionally or never?
>   Yes/0 points

Do you take them once or twice annually for short courses of fewer than 2 weeks?
>   Yes/5 points

Do you take them 3–4 times each year, or single courses over 4 weeks?
>   Yes/10 points

STEROIDS

Do you use a steroid inhaler (e.g. Becotide) for asthma on a regular basis?

    Yes/10 points

    No/0 points

Do you regularly take steroid drugs (e.g. prednisolone) for arthritis or other problems?

    Yes/10 points

    No/0 points

Have you had more than one cortisone injection within the last 12 months?

    Yes/10 points

    No/0 points

DIABETES

Have you mild diabetes controlled by diet?

    Yes/0 points

Have you diabetes (Type II) controlled by drugs?

    Yes/5 points

Have you diabetes (Type I) controlled by insulin injections?

    Yes/10 points

STRESS

Over the previous 5 years has your stress load been:

    Trivial/0 points

    Average/5 points

    Severe/10 points

INFECTIONS

Are you prone to frequent infections (e.g. colds, flu, chest, etc.)?

    Yes/10 points

    No/0 points

PREGNANCY
Have you ever been pregnant?
   No/0 points
   Once/5 points
   Twice or more/10 points

HYPOTHYROID
Do you regularly take thyroxine for an underactive thyroid?
   Yes/10 points
   No/0 points

STOMACH AND DUODENAL ULCERS
Do you regularly take drugs to reduce digestive acid (e.g. Losec)?
   No/0 points
   Yes/10 points

Part 2 – Symptoms
The list below includes the major symptoms caused by candidiasis. Score as follows for each symptom.

1   No, you do not suffer this symptom/0 points
2   You suffer this symptom, but only mildly and occasionally/5 points
3   This symptom is chronic and severe/10 points

- Abdominal bloating and/or pain
- Chronic diarrhoea/constipation
- Intestinal gas and belching
- Hiatus hernia (heartburn)
- Haemorrhoids
- Pruritus – itching skin in groin, buttock or vagina
- Rashes, eczema or allergic skin reactions
- Fungal problems around nails e.g. athlete's foot
- Adverse reaction to tobacco smoke, petrol fumes, household cleaners, perfume, pesticides, etc.

- Frequent bladder infections
- Vaginal or oral thrush
- Period pain or PMS
- Bladder frequency with burning or poor control
- Bad breath or body odour
- Ear infections
- Throat infections
- Rhinitis (all-year-round hay fever-type symptoms)
- Nasal congestion, poor sense of smell
- Muscle weakness, pain or stiffness
- Tendency for joints to swell
- Fatigue
- Food intolerance or sensitivity
- Poor concentration, poor short-term memory
- Depression, anxiety or irritability
- Cravings for sweet foods, alcohol, chocolate, vinegar, bread, cereals, cakes or biscuits
- Regular headaches
- Excessive hunger, being anxious or irritable if meals are delayed
- Feeling lethargic, irritable and anxious on waking
- Poor libido
- Symptoms worsened by damp or humid weather conditions
- 'Floaters' in the eyes, with poor night vision

Scoring

200 points or over	It is probable that you are suffering from candidiasis.
100–200 points	It is possible that your symptoms may be caused by candidiasis.
100 points or fewer	It is unlikely that candidiasis is your problem.

This questionnaire offers useful diagnostic clues to identify candidiasis. However, laboratory testing can provide further information on the existence and status of any candida overgrowth.

Testing for Candidiasis

Candida Antibody Blood Test

For some years I regularly requested a candida antibody (or antigen) blood test to assist candida diagnosis. However, after several years of use I realized that *all* my patients tested appeared to have developed an immune response to candida (unfortunately, the antibodies can persist even after the candidiasis is cleared). This factor, coupled with the test's failure to demonstrate the degree of severity of the overgrowth, have rendered this particular test unreliable in my opinion.

Comprehensive Digestive Stool Analysis

This test is done by the Great Smokies Diagnostic Laboratory in North Carolina, US. It provides, among other results, a dysbiosis index, a beneficial bacteria rating, and a candida 'score'. Although the test costs around £120, it provides a comprehensive view of intestinal health, including the current status of any candida overgrowth.

Gut Fermentation Test

This is a blood test that measures various blood alcohols after the patient has taken 1 gm of glucose (as any brewer knows, yeast can convert sugar into alcohol).

My protocol when faced with a potential candidiasis patient is as follows:

1 Request a Gut Permeability (leaky gut) test
2 Symptom assessment
3 Stool analysis or gut fermentation test (if a 'leaky gut' is confirmed)
4 Treatment.

The value of interpreting a diagnostic test is that improvement can be seen and assessed without total reliance on subjective symptom changes. Symptom changes do not always reflect or parallel actual health changes. If a patient has several health problems, it can be difficult to assess progress. It is at such times that actual test results can be re-assuring and helpful. They can also offer a guide to required supplement dosages and possible prognosis.

Treatment of Candidiasis

The control and treatment of candida overgrowth falls into four stages:

Stage 1   Avoidance of drugs and hormones that can cause candidiasis

Stage 2   Following an anti-candida diet and lifestyle

Stage 3   Taking steps to improve your digestive and immune efficiency

Stage 4   Taking supplements to minimize nutrient deficiencies, to kill off or reduce the candida colony, and to repopulate the gastrointestinal tract with the beneficial bacteria that normally police and control the yeast population.

Stage 1

To treat candidiasis, you must try to reduce, or if possible eliminate completely, the various hormones and drugs that are known to cause it. These include steroids, antacids, antibiotics and the contraceptive pill. (It is of course necessary to discuss any changes regarding medication with your doctor.)

Stage 2

Diet
An ideal anti-candida diet should adhere to two main recommendations:

1 Avoid foods and drinks with a yeast or mould content.
2 Avoid sugar-rich foods, and keep carbohydrates to a minimum. (Yeast feeds on sugar!)

There are many different anti-candida diets advocated by various authors and practitioners. On page 118 you will find the dietary guidelines I recommend for my patients.

Stage 3

Digestive and Immune Efficiency
Any imbalance in the digestive enzymes and stomach acidity encourages candida growth, as does immune exhaustion. Therefore, these two areas may need to be addressed.

The pancreactic enzymes play a special role. They break down proteins, but also assist in the control of parasites in the intestine, which include bacteria, protozoa (single-cell parasites), intestinal worms and yeasts. (See Chapter 7 for more details on digestive enzyme use.)

A healthy, efficient immune system is essential for candida control. Many factors can compromise and weaken our immune system:

Undernourishment, including low protein diets and vitamin
and mineral deficiencies
High-sugar diets (it has been suggested that excessive sugar
reduces the availability of Vitamin C in the body)
Obesity with raised levels of blood fats (triglycerides
and cholesterol)
Alcohol
Antibiotics, steroids and various hormones
Diabetes
Anaemia
Hypothyroidism (underactive thyroid)
Stress
Cancer
Chemicals in our environment and food

Treating the Immune System
Many vitamins, minerals, plant remedies and nutrients are recommended to support the immune system. These include vitamin A, vitamin B complex, vitamin C and propolis, astragalus, calendula, echinacea, goldenseal, hydrastis, olive leaf extract, garlic, liquorice, borage, comfrey, sage, wild yam, Siberian ginseng and wild indigo, the essential fatty acids (Omega 3 and 6), selenium, iron (when deficient), zinc and calcium. The amino acid (protein component) glutathione can aid the immune response and assist allergies, inflammation and pain.

Stage 4

Nutritional Supplements to Treat Candidiasis
Caprylic acid, an extract from coconut, assists control of candida overgrowth by encouraging the beneficial intestinal flora. Other

plant remedies frequently seen in anti-candida formulations are Pau d'Arco, aloe vera, and grapefruit seed extract.

PROBIOTICS
This name describes the friendly gut bacteria. Unlike antibiotics, which reduce the beneficial bacteria, the probiotics replenish them. Natural live yoghourt should contain probiotics.

Fortunately, the three 'good' bacteria – namely *Lactobacillus acidophilus*, *Lactobacillus bulgaricus*, and *Lactobacillus bifidus* – can all be taken in capsule form.

To emphasize the importance of the lactobacilli to human health, it may be of value to look at the benefits they can offer when taken as supplements:

1   They control unfriendly, hostile yeasts such as candida albicans.
2   They are involved in the metabolism of certain B vitamins.
3   They have a cholesterol-lowering role.
4   By producing the enzyme lactase, they beneficially influence lactose (milk sugar) digestion.

VITAMINS AND MINERALS
Nutritional therapy to treat candida overgrowth usually includes the following minerals and vitamins:

Vitamin B Complex (yeast-free)
Selenium
Biotin
Zinc
Vitamin C + bioflavonoids
Magnesium
Vitamin B_5
Iron
Vitamin E
Vitamin A (Beta Carotene)

EXSPORE™

When prescribing for candida patients, I usually favour this supplement. Supplied by Nutri (see Resources), it combines anti-fungal plant remedies and probiotics.

I have listed its contents below in order to give you an idea of its value and complexity.

Caprylic Acid, Zinc, Molydenum, Garlic, Aloe Vera, Pau d'Arco, Tillandsia, Beet, Cinnamon, Thyme, Basil, Manganese, Citrus Seed Extract, Cloves, N-Acetyl Glucosamine, Goldenseal, Niacin, Oregano Oil, Co-Enzyme, Q-10, Lactobacillus Bulgaricus, Lactobacillus Bifidus

Conclusion

The successful treatment of candida albicans is rarely simple or rapid. When an overgrowth develops, it is usually a product of a variety of adverse factors ranging from prolonged antibiotic use, thyroid or adrenal exhaustion to poor nutrition. Unfortunately, I find that just as candidiasis can produce a number of symptoms, it can develop as a result of a number of causes.

Dietary discipline, lifestyle changes where indicated, and appropriate supplementation can usually improve intestinal health and remove another common cause of excess weight.

Anna's Story

Consultation

Anna's problems began in her mouth. Following serial dental abscesses nine years earlier, which were treated with broad-spectrum antibiotics, she developed the symptoms of chronic candida overgrowth. When she consulted me she recounted an unhappy story of virtually non-stop stomach discomfort and stomach bloating after meals, chronic diarrhoea, vaginal thrush and cystitis. In addition she was overweight, tired and forgetful, with a non-existent libido. Perhaps not surprisingly, she was also very depressed.

Anna was 54 years old and had passed through menopause two years earlier. Her mother had had diabetes. At 5 ft 3 in (160 cm) tall her weight was excessive at 178 lb (81 kg), giving her a BMI of 31, just into the 'obese' range. Her only current treatment was self-prescribed and included a low-dose vitamin C capsule, 2–3 garlic capsules each day, and a multi-vitamin-mineral formula.

Tests

I am sometimes tempted to request a standard profile of tests for all my candidiasis patients. However the cost, coupled with the need for an individual assessment for each patient, make any such standard approach unrealistic.

Although Anna's problems stemmed from systemic candidiasis, she also experienced chronic stomach symptoms including bloating, possibly caused by a reduced stomach acid level, slow stomach emptying or generally inefficient and delayed food digestion.

With this in mind I requested a gut-fermentation profile, a gut permeability test, and a gastrogram.

Gastrogram

This test requires the patient to attend a laboratory in London (Biolab). A small capsule is swallowed by the patient and then signals from the three zinc electrodes contained in the capsule provide information on stomach acidity (pH), stomach-emptying speed, and pancreatic enzyme levels. This valuable test does not cause any discomfort to the patient and takes approximately 45 minutes. The capsule is subsequently passed and does not need to be recovered.

Results

Anna's gut fermentation profile showed elevated ethanol consistent with a marked yeast overgrowth. The gut permeability test confirmed a 'leaky gut' with an increased permeability of six of the eleven molecules of the polyethylene glycol.

The gastrogram showed 'normal' pancreatic enzyme function and 'normal' stomach emptying. However, Anna's stomach acidity was very low. When gastric acid secretion is low, this is termed *hypochlorhydria*. We so often tend to associate stomach symptoms with an 'acid stomach' when, for many of us, the opposite is true. (In studies with women over 50 years, up to 40% had severely low stomach acid levels.) The stomach acid is mainly responsible for the digestion of proteins. If this digestion is incomplete or delayed as a result of hypochlorhydria, the production of vital enzymes, hormones and other substances is compromised.

The acidity of the normal stomach when digesting food is around pH3, and neutral is pH7 (anything below pH7 indicates acidity; anything above pH7 is alkaline). When groups of normal (symptom-free) men and women were tested for their fasting stomach acid levels, for the men hypochlorhydria was found in 29%, and for the women 61%.

Treatment

When intestinal permeability is increased (leaky gut syndrome), it is essential to normalize or repair the gut lining before taking supplements. If this is not done, the absorption of the supplements will be inefficient and incomplete.

L. Glutamine

This amino acid (protein) is prescribed to assist leaky gut repair. I have found it remarkably and predictably effective in normalizing permeability. I frequently request follow-up tests to assess permeability, and the results usually show normal absorption after 6–8 weeks of treatment. The dosage of L. Glutamine I recommend in these cases is 3,000 mg daily taken between meals.

When Anna's absorption was improved, I prescribed a course of Exspore™ to reduce the candida activity, and advised her to follow a low-sugar, low-carbohydrate and yeast-free diet.

To assist her protein digestion and resulting stomach fullness, I recommended that Anna took a two-phase digestive enzyme containing hydrochloric acid (betaine HCL) and pepsin. This is called Hypo-D, and is formulated as follows:

1st Phase (in Stomach)	2nd Phase (in Duodenum)
Betaine HCL	Pancreatin
L-Glutamine Acid HCL	Pancrelipase
Pepsin	Amylase
Papain	Ox Bile
	Bromelain
	Parotid

Within a period of six months Anna, was virtually symptom-free. After the first two months she'd no longer needed the supplements for the stomach acidity and leaky gut, but was on a low-maintenance dose of Exspore™ and the diet to control the candidiasis. Her weight had gone down to 148 lb (67 kg) with a BMI of 26, and her vitality was around 75% of normal. She was obviously converting food to energy (rather than fat) more efficiently.

Anna's mood was also improved. I so often find that depression is linked to fatigue. It is very rare to meet a depressed person who is not fatigued. I advised Anna at our last meeting to contact me if she was ever again prescribed antibiotics. There are alternatives available that do not upset the delicate balance of intestinal bacteria and yeast. If antibiotics are absolutely essential (as with certain dental and middle-ear conditions, meningitis, etc.), it is always wise to take supplementary probiotics, the B vitamins and anti-candidiasis supplements as a safeguard.

Chapter Summary

1 Candida albicans is a yeast strain that lives in the human digestive tract, being controlled by beneficial bacteria.

2 Although harmless when controlled, if it increases and overgrows it can cause a leaky gut, Irritable Bowel Syndrome (IBS), overweight, fatigue, food intolerances and other symptoms.

3 Many factors can cause candida to increase, including antibiotics, stress, a high-sugar diet, various prescription drugs and alcohol.

4 If candida changes to a fungal type, a leaky gut may result, with IBS, food intolerances and immune stress. Tests are available to measure leaky gut and the presence of an overgrowth of candida.

5 A yeast- and sugar-free diet is recommended to treat candida, coupled with probiotics and specific nutritional and plant supplements.

6 Yeast imbalance can lead to a range of symptoms, but when these are addressed you can improve your general health and lose weight successfully.

Dietary Guidelines for Candida Control

Avoid

Sugar in all forms and all bread and flour products (e.g. cake and biscuits), EXCEPT yeast-free unleavened bread and rice cakes
Alcohol in all forms
Citrus juices, unless freshly squeezed
Malt drinks
Nuts, unless freshly cracked and in season
Cereals containing added vitamins and malt

All dried fruits (unless guaranteed yeast-free)

Fungi, mushrooms and moulds

Foods containing monosodium glutamate (E621)

All types of vinegar including balsamic, cider, malt and grape-based varieties

Buttermilk and yoghourt with added vitamins

Anything fried in breadcrumbs (e.g. fish fingers)

Meat extracts (OXO, Marmite, etc.)

Hamburgers, sausages, smoked fish and meats

Condiments and pickles, salad dressings, sauerkraut, olives, chillies, etc.

Blue cheeses (e.g. Stilton)

Any vitamins or minerals unless they are from a non-yeast source (e.g. rice)

When buying meat try to obtain antibiotic and hormone-free meat from a local farm shop or similar specialist country supplier. Pork is best avoided.

If possible avoid damp atmospheres and old buildings that may support moulds and rot e.g. cellars, old clothes and books.

All fruits and vegetables should be as fresh as possible, and well washed before use.

Drink still mineral water only.

Use only freshly laundered towels, damp bath towels encourage mould growth.

If you know or suspect that you are sensitive to certain foods, these should be avoided. Food allergies or intolerances can weaken the immune system and encourage yeast growth.

CHAPTER SIX

Food Allergies and Your Weight

Food allergies and sensitivities usually involve inappropriate – and certainly unwanted – responses to common foods. Even the foods you eat every day can cause unpleasant symptoms, including weight gain.

Food Allergy

What is sometimes referred to as a 'classical allergy' describes an immediate and severe reaction to a specific food. A well-known example is the severe reaction some people experience when eating peanuts. With children, the resulting anaphylactic shock can be life-threatening, often requiring casualty treatment. This type of reaction causes a particular antibody or immunoglobulin response. There are five classes of immunoglobulins. The one that triggers an immediate allergic response is termed IgE. Others in the group include IgA, IgD, IgC and IgM.

When IgE was identified in the early 1960s, it was recognized as the chief culprit in classical allergies. The RAST (radio-allergo-sorbent test) developed to help identify allergies shows raised blood levels of IgE in many patients who suffer a sudden and often violent reaction to common foods. However, many patients do not show a high IgE, and their responses to foods were sometimes delayed for up to two to three days. With this type of delayed reaction, it is not always easy to identify the suspect food or foods.

Food Sensitivity

The terms 'sensitivity' or 'intolerance' are considered more appropriate names for this type of delayed response to certain foods, as it is not a classic allergy and does not involve a raised IgE level. This type of reaction does, however, lead to raised levels of another antibody, IgG. When a patient's blood makes contact with specific foods, it is this type of reaction or intolerance that causes the many subtle and varied symptoms associated with food sensitivities. These include weight gain. The symptoms are sometimes defined as 'stress-induced' by those who do not accept that foods can cause symptoms. The test that is used to recognize such sensitivities is known as the ELISA (enzyme-linked immuno-absorbent assay). I frequently request this test, as it only requires a very small finger prick blood sample, making it an ideal test for small children (and nervous adults). The results, which fall into six levels of response (depending on sensitivity), are approximately 85% reliable and very useful to identify hidden or masked food sensitivities. (See Resources – York Nutritional Laboratory.)

Symptoms of Food Sensitivities

The symptoms that you may be suffering from a food sensitivity include:

weight gain
IBS (Irritable Bowel Syndrome)-type symptoms

constipation
eczema
joint pain
catarrh and sinusitis
anxiety and depression
headaches (including migraine)
fatigue
fluid retention
hyperactivity in children
muscle pain and stiffness
poor concentration and short-term memory.

Readers will note that many of these symptoms parallel those of mild hypothyroidism (see Chapter 9), giving a clue to the many problems that are involved in diagnosing the causes of such symptoms as headaches, fatigue and excess weight.

Are You Food Sensitive?

Later in this chapter I shall describe the simple tests on offer to help you to answer this question. Meanwhile, this questionnaire will begin to provide you with important information. For every 'Yes' answer, give yourself 5 points.

1 Do you feel at your worst on rising?
2 Do you experience muscle and joint pain on waking?
3 Are you unnaturally tired after a meal?
4 Did you as a child suffer any of the following: throat infections, eczema, asthma, sinusitis, glue ear?
5 Do you have a strong urge to eat certain foods such as eggs, milk, bread?
6 Do you experience fullness after meals, or suffer from regular diarrhoea or constipation?

7 Do you suffer from unexplained skin rashes, eczema or urticaria (hives)?

8 Do you regularly have dark circles beneath your eyes, even when you are not tired?

9 Do you retain fluid, with puffy ankles (and tight shoes) at the end of the day, with a weight increase of 1–2 pounds over the course of the day?

10 Has your weight increased over the previous 12 months, even with the same diet and activities?

11 Do you experience regular, unexplained headaches?

12 Do you sometimes feel confused, 'woolly-headed' and forgetful?

Scoring

0–20   You are an unlikely candidate for a food intolerance diagnosis

20–35   A diagnosis of food intolerance is a possibility and further testing is recommended

35–60   A diagnosis of food intolerance is a probability and further testing is essential to confirm which foods are involved

Gary's Story

Consultation

Gary was a 41-year-old accountant. He had tried many different diets in an attempt to reduce his weight. At the time he came to see me he weighed 232 lb (105 kg) – at 6 ft 3 in (190 cm) this gave him a BMI of 29 (just under 'obese'). He was a typical 'yo-yo' dieter. Any restricted special diet usually resulted in an initial loss of 6–8 lb (3–4 kg) in the first 10 days. The weight then plateaued, and after 3–4 weeks Gary despaired, returned to his usual diet and replaced the weight lost in 7–10 days.

Upon questioning Gary, however, it soon became obvious that excess weight was not his only health problem.

Up until six years previously he had enjoyed an excellent state of health and weight, being 190 lb (86 kg). But then he had suffered a severe dental abscess following root canal work which required two courses of antibiotics to clear the infection.

Within one week of completing the second course of antibiotics, Gary knew that something was not right. He developed stomach fullness and discomfort after meals, a persistent dull morning headache and non-stop rhinitis (itchy, runny nose). Gary had suffered mild seasonal hay fever for many years. This usually caused several weeks of sneezing in May and June. Now the rhinitis was constant, however, and made much worse by smoky atmospheres, household dust and traffic fumes. He felt worst on rising, and was so congested that he was unable to breathe clearly through his nose until around lunch time. His non-stop sniffing was a source of irritation to his wife and work colleagues. In addition to the above symptoms, Gary was tired. On waking he felt thick-headed and sluggish. In short, Gary had not felt well since the course of antibiotics he'd had six years earlier.

As discussed in Chapter 5, modern broad-spectrum antibiotics kill the beneficial bacteria as well as the 'bad' bacteria in our systems. This can cause systemic candida in the intestines which can lead to a 'leaky gut' and food intolerances. Food intolerances can in turn cause fluid retention and a general depression of our metabolism.

Treatment

Tests confirmed that Gary did have a leaky gut and a moderate candida problem. These two conditions were treated, and a subsequent gut permeability test confirmed that the gut was normal. I then requested a food intolerance blood test or ELISA.

Gary's test showed a severe reaction to cows' milk and eggs, and a mild response to yeast and wheat.

I asked Gary to write down everything he ate or drank over the next three days. This showed me that he was having milk (in butter and cheese, etc.) every day, and egg or egg products four or five days out of seven. I therefore advised him to avoid cows' milk and eggs for six weeks, and to eat foods containing wheat or yeast no more than once each week.

When the six weeks were completed I prescribed a short course of pillules containing egg and milk in homoeopathic (trace) potencies. Gary took these twice daily before beginning a rotation diet plan (see below) to reintroduce eggs and cows' milk. These tiny amounts of the suspect foods serve to condition the digestive system to accept the foods, but without the patient's symptoms of intolerance resurfacing. (It is essential not to give sensitive patients any homoeopathic remedies that are formulated with a lactose base; instead, fructose-based remedies should be used.)

After a further rotation plan on eggs and milk for four weeks, Gary was able to eat all the foods he'd reacted to on the ELISA, on a daily basis. I also advised him to take plant enzymes before each meal to aid his digestion (see Chapter 7).

Gary's symptoms improved after two weeks of avoiding the milk and eggs; he awoke refreshed and able to breathe clearly through his nose. Without any changes to his diet except the programme outlined above, he slowly began to lose weight. He now felt fit enough to walk for 20 minutes before work each morning, and to swim two to three times weekly.

Four months after his initial consultation, Gary's weight was down to 212 lb (96 kg); two months later he weighed 198 lb (90 kg) with a resulting BMI of just below 25.

Conclusion

Gary's case serves to highlight the common link between overweight and ill-health. The antibiotics had impaired his digestive efficiency, leading to fatigue, fluid retention and many other symptoms. Digestive enzymes assisted Gary's conversion of food to energy, and the daily exercise boosted his flagging metabolic rate. His weight only began to normalize, however, after his food intolerances were corrected.

Testing for Food Intolerance

The Pulse Test

In 1956 an American doctor named Arthur F. Coca wrote a small book entitled *The Pulse Test*. This book described a very simple method of diagnosing food sensitivities based on the fact that our pulse accelerates when we eat foods that we react to (allergens). Dr Coca held the controversial view that, as the normal pulse rate is not predictably affected by ordinary activity and emotions, any frequent variations of the pulse rate are probably caused by food intolerances. First, other causes of a temporary increase in the pulse rate need to be excluded, including overheating, stress, exertion and infection. Dr Coca described this concept as follows: 'The pulse then may be considered a dependable first watchdog of our health-citadel, telling us promptly whenever we are in possibly injurious contact with our allergic enemies.'

Method

1 As environmental allergens exist for many people, it is essential not to smoke while pulse testing is being used.
2 The pulse is checked for 60 seconds several times a day, as follows:
   a) upon waking
   b) a few minutes before each meal
   c) 30, 60 and 90 minutes after each meal
   d) upon retiring

3 All checks are made while you are seated (except the check made on waking, which should be done before you sit up). The procedure involves a total of 14 checks daily (assuming you eat three meals a day).
4 Make a note of all foods eaten and all drinks. This needs to be quite detailed.
5 Do pulse checks for a minimum of three days.

Assuming that the pulse confirms a reaction to food, you can follow this up with single-food checks. This is best done at the weekend. The procedure involves eating a single food every hour after the resting pulse check on waking. As many as 30 foods can be tested in this way over two days.

Interpreting the Pulse Test Results
As with all tests, a baseline 'normal' needs to be identified. Your pulse rate can be complicated by nondietary factors or triggers. These can include house dust, cosmetics, newspaper print, cleaning materials, etc.

The female hormones have also been known to influence the pulse rate pre-menstrually and at mid-cycle during ovulation (around day 14 of your menstrual cycle). For these reasons, women should not try the pulse test at these times in their cycle.

Over the initial three days of pulse testing, the lowest and the highest counts are recorded. The optimum range for human pulse measurement is 16 beats. In other words, if over the three days you record a lowest figure of, say, 58 beats per minute and a highest of perhaps 72 beats, this provides a difference of 14 beats. You are therefore unlikely to be a food sensitive.

If, however, your count reveals a difference of 24 beats per minute, a food sensitivity would be worth investigating further.

Once your normal range – that is, the difference between your lowest and fastest pulse rate has been established, it is not difficult to recognize pulse increases caused by food sensitivity.

When it has been established that your pulse rate increases above your 'normal' maximum rate after eating, the next step is the 'single-food test'.

The Single-Food Test

The object of this test is to identify the foods that you are sensitive to by pulse testing after eating them, one at a time.

Procedure – Day 1
Take your pulse on waking (while you are still in bed), and again immediately before your first food. Check your pulse 30 minutes after the test food and again 60 minutes after. Immediately after the 60-minute pulse count, you eat another single food. You measure your pulse throughout the day on this basis. A record must be kept of the foods eaten and the pulse counts. Suspect foods will accelerate your pulse rate, 'safe' foods will not influence it. As mixed meals can mask the response in terms of pulse rate and the symptoms, testing foods one at a time is important in determining the true culprit(s).

Examples of single foods you might want to test are listed below. This list includes the most common food allergens.

NB
Do not test foods that you know cause symptoms, or foods that disagree with you. It is also not necessary to test foods that you very rarely eat.

Many foods belong to large 'families' – for example, cabbage is a member of the mustard family, which includes broccoli, Brussels sprouts, Chinese leaves, horseradish, kohlrabi, kale, cress, radish, rapeseed, mustard, watercress and turnip. So the testing of perhaps 25–30 foods and drinks over a two-day period means that you are in reality testing upwards of 200+ foods, belonging to different food 'families'.

So, assuming you consume these foods and drinks on a regular basis – that is, at least once a week – your initial test programme could include the following:

Cows' milk	Bread	Potato	Prune
Goats' milk	Rice	Cabbage	Strawberry
Soya milk	Sugar	Lettuce	Melon
Coffee (black)	Chocolate	Mushroom	Orange
Egg white	Beef	Carrot	Apple
Egg yolk	Chicken	Onion	Pineapple
	Prawn	Corn	Blackcurrant
	Salmon		
	Tuna		
	Cod		

When compiling such a chart, the chief drawback of elimination-reintroduction testing becomes apparent – time. This becomes a significant factor when avoiding and testing as many as 20 foods and drinks. Your list will include the common foods that many people are sensitive to (e.g. milk, wheat, coffee) plus your own personal 'frequent' foods. You will soon have 15–20 foods to test. As you need to allow 3 clear days between each 'test' food, you can only test 7 foods in 4 weeks. A list of 20 foods will therefore involve nearly 3 months testing! Nevertheless, this type of testing for food sensitivity is seen by many practitioners as the benchmark for food intolerance testing.

The Results
Pulse testing should not be seen as a definitive guide to your food sensitivities, but it can be a useful self-assessment first step in recognizing the hidden causes of your symptoms.

I shall now look at other methods of food intolerance detection.

The Elimination/Provocation (Reintroduction) Method

This provides a simple, effective way to assess your sensitivity to common foods.

If you have a suspicion that your food is contributing to your symptoms, then eliminate all the common problem foods, plus any particular foods you may suspect, from your diet for a minimum of two weeks. If after the two-week avoidance of suspect foods your symptoms improve, then it is very likely that you have a food sensitivity. You can then reintroduce the foods one at a time, and those foods that cause a return of your symptoms are the foods that you are sensitive to. This method works in part because your symptom-response to a particular food can be significantly increased following a period of avoidance.

Foods to Avoid
With elimination-reintroduction testing it is essential, if the method is to work, for you to experience symptom-relief following the initial two-week food avoidance. If symptom-relief is not experienced, there are two possible causes:

1 The offending foods have not been avoided and they are still therefore causing symptoms.
2 You do not have any food intolerances and the causes of your symptoms lie elsewhere.

To ensure that the food-elimination phase is beneficial and effective, the following guidelines need to be considered when you draw up your list of foods to avoid.

1 Avoid foods which in your experience can cause symptoms. Also avoid any foods for which you experience a craving.
2 Avoid cows' milk and all cows' milk products including butter, cream, yoghourt and cheese.

3 Avoid wheat and all sources of wheat (wheat and cows' milk
   always feature at the top of the list of food sensitivities).
   Wheat occurs in a huge range of foods. These include bread,
   cakes, biscuits, pasta, pastry, some breakfast cereals, etc.
   Many processed foods contain wheat, sometimes defined as
   'edible starch'. You need to be conscientious about reading
   labels, or simply avoid processed foods and any doubtful
   mixes.
4 Just to complete your food avoidance list, it is also advisable
   to avoid any food or drink that you consume every day, such
   as tea, coffee, eggs, orange juice, potatoes, wine. (Foods and
   drinks that are consumed frequently, are more likely to cause
   symptoms than those eaten only occasionally.)

Replacement Foods
The next obvious consideration is what to have in place of the foods
that you are avoiding for two weeks.

Here is a list of optional alternatives:

Foods to be avoided	Alternatives
Cows' milk	Goats' milk, cheese and yoghourt
	Sheep's milk cheese and yoghourt
	Soya milk and yoghourt
	Rice and coconut milk
Wheat	Wheat-free bread and cereal
	Rice products, oat and corn cereals, rice cakes and biscuits, rye bread and biscuits
Pasta (durum wheat)	Rice pasta
Coffee and tea	Dandelion coffee, herbal teas, fruit teas, various coffee substitutes

Remember, this elimination or avoidance stage only lasts two
weeks!

Reintroduction (Provocation)

Assuming that during the two weeks' avoidance you are experiencing some symptom-relief, you can begin to reintroduce the suspect foods and assess your responses to them. This is known as the *reintroduction* or *provocation* stage.

It is important to realize that eliminating suspect foods can heighten your sensitivity to the foods when they are reintroduced into your diet. The foods that you have been avoiding for two weeks must be reintroduced one at a time. If symptoms return (e.g. fatigue, depression, headache, rhinitis, diarrhoea, stomach discomfort, etc.) within three days of reintroducing a food, avoid that food once again and test another food. The reaction to a suspect food can occur up to 72 hours after eating, hence the essential three-day delay before retesting.

If you feel symptom-free after the three days, it is very unlikely that you are sensitive to the particular food tested. Continue to work through your list, taking note of what seem to be 'problem' foods and 'safe' foods.

Though time-consuming and calling for real diligence, this method is seen by many practitioners as the benchmark for food intolerance testing.

ELISA Testing

For those who can't face the tedium of food avoidance and provocation testing or pulse assessment, the ELISA test may be the answer.

ELISA stands for enzyme-linked immuno-absorbent assay. It is a blood test during which a very small amount of whole blood (a pin-prick is sufficient) is taken and sent to the laboratory. (The ease of sample-taking makes this an ideal test for babies and children.) The blood is presented to a panel of foods (usually a minimum of 40 foods) and the immune complexes (IgGs) that develop as a result of the contact are measured. If your blood shows such complexes, this confirms that the food concerned is toxic to your blood.

The reactions are graded into six levels of severity, ranging from 'no reaction' to 'avoid'.

Unfortunately, the level of the test result-grading does not always parallel symptom severity. However, as a general rule, the higher the blood reaction, the more likely a food will cause your symptoms.

Many of the 40 foods tested belong to large food families, so in reality the ELISA can be seen to 'cover' 200 or more foods.

The Causes of Food Sensitivity

The exact cause of food sensitivities is still a subject of speculation and dispute within the world of nutrition and medicine.

The concept of food intolerance has never fitted comfortably into orthodox medical diagnoses. Adverse reactions to food have a tendency to involve several body systems. An intolerance to a specific food may cause symptoms as diverse as indigestion, muscle pain, headaches, depression and poor skin and hair, all at the same time in the same patient. So many symptoms can bewilder a doctor – when a diagnostic pigeon-hole cannot be found, the diagnosis of 'stress' or 'depression' is often offered as the most appropriate.

Symptoms that are caused by common foods are frequently defined as 'functional'. This describes a health disorder that does not need to include disease or damage, but is simply a result of inefficiency, sensitivity or imbalance in one or more of the body systems. Unfortunately the diagnostic tests aimed at discovering, for example, the cause of indigestion (e.g. gastroscopies and scans) are designed to identify structural changes (e.g. cancer and ulcers) and not subtle imbalances in the stomach acid level or digestive enzyme status.

The Gluten Puzzle

Gluten intolerance is known as coeliac disease. This is termed an inborn error of metabolism (something you are born with), and involves an inability to absorb the gluten in certain cereals. This malabsorption causes many symptoms including diarrhoea, abdominal distention, muscle cramping and fatigue, also weight changes and flatulence.

Gluten is a protein complex found in wheat, oats, rye and barley. It is the gluten (or gliadin) in wheat and other grains which gives dough its tough elastic property. It is worth noting the term 'wheat-free' seen on some food product labels is not always the same as 'gluten-free'. It may be that your reaction to wheat is in fact caused by one of the proteins found in the grain.

If it is found when testing that you have reacted to several cereals (excluding corn and rice), gluten-intolerance should be considered.

A simple blood test named the gliadin-antibody test is seen as a reliable test for this intolerance. This test is 98% accurate.

Avoidance
Elimination of gluten from one's diet is far from easy, but eating gluten-free products and grains (corn and rice) is the only answer to symptom relief.

Lactose Intolerance

Lactose is the sugar found in the milk of all mammals (except seals). The cause of the lactose intolerance is a deficiency or defect in the enzyme *lactase*. Lactase normally breaks lactose down into the simple sugars glucose and galactose.

Although usually an inherited abnormality, lactose intolerance can also develop following stomach surgery (partial gastrectomy), as a result of disease of the small intestine, malnutrition, and taking some types of antibiotics.

Testing for Lactose Intolerance
The chief test is a Lactose Tolerance Test. This simple but rather unpleasant test involves the patient attending the laboratory after a

12- to 14-hour water-only fast. After an initial measurement of the patient's blood glucose, they are given 50 gm of soluble lactose to drink. With normal lactose levels, the lactose, when consumed, will be split into glucose and galactose, with a subsequent predictable rise in the blood glucose level. This increase in blood glucose is assessed with a further blood glucose check over a 2-hour period. If the patient's lactase is deficient or absent, the rise in their blood glucose is minimal or absent. A further confirmation of lactose intolerance is that the symptoms themselves (abdominal discomfort, acute diarrhoea, nausea) can develop during the test. These may be severe enough cause the test to be terminated.

Avoidance of all milk and milk-containing products can lead to symptom-relief, but this is not a lasting answer. Taking milk-digesting enzymes and lactase tablets just before eating foods or drinks that contain milk is a satisfactory solution.

The symptom benefits achieved with enzyme use are diagnostically useful and can avoid the need for lactose tolerance testing. Most of my patients who have lactose intolerance avoid milk at home, when they are in control of their food selection and content, and make use of lactase tablets when eating out or on holiday. Milk that contains lactose is now available at certain stores. The symptoms of lactose intolerance include abdominal bloating and pain, nausea, diarrhoea, stomach cramps and flatulence. All of which can develop after ingesting milk or milk products.

PROLACTAZYME FORTE™
Various supplement suppliers include a milk-digesting enzyme formula in their product catalogue. However, I have found that Prolactazyme Forte™ by Biocare (see Resources) is very effective for treating lactose intolerance.

The ingredients include:

Rennin (vegetable source)	Lactase	Bromelain
Lipase	Papain	Amylase
MicroCell	Acidophilus	Lactobacillus bulgaricus

Liquid lactase is also available for children.

Katy's Story

Consultation

Katy, 28, had tried everything to lose weight. She visited a local gym at least four times a week for an hour and a half each time. Her exercise regime included a circuit on the equipment followed by a swim and a sauna. Her work as an insurance agent was sedentary, but in addition to her gym activities she enjoyed coastal walking with her partner. They usually managed to walk 8–10 miles each weekend.

Katy's diet was excellent. Being a lover of Greece and Southern France, she had developed a taste for Mediterranean food. She therefore ate a lot of salads and fruit, fish, cheese and pasta, with chicken and, occasionally, lamb. She drank around 20 units of wine each week, and smoked 20 cigarettes a week.

Katy was 5 ft 4 in (163 cm) and weighed 157 lb (71 kg), giving her a BMI of 27 (well into the 'overweight' range of 25–30). Katy had been overweight since puberty.

When I am consulted by overweight patients, after the initial facts and figures have been established my next question is always, 'Do you feel well, or do you have other health problems aside from your weight?' Symptoms can supply valuable clues to lead to the cause or causes of overweight.

Symptoms

Katy's symptoms included frequent diarrhoea and nausea, dizziness after main meals, and chronic heartburn and stomach fullness after eating. None of these symptoms was severe, however, and Katy had never sought treatment for them, although they had been with her since childhood. She admitted to being far more concerned over her stubborn overweight.

I concluded that Katy was not metabolizing her food efficiently. This suggested an enzyme deficiency, low stomach acidity (hypochlorhydria – see page 143), or a single or multiple food intolerance. All these problems can result in fluid retention and increased body weight. I therefore requested a gastric function test (gastrogram – see page 115) and gut permeability profile (to check for leaky gut syndrome). All the results returned as 'normal', except for a borderline pancreatic enzyme level of 65%. Katy's stomach emptying speed, stomach acidity and gut absorption were all quite normal.

The remaining 'option' was the possibility that Katy was experiencing symptoms of food intolerance. I discussed the various methods used to identify possible food sensitivities, and Katy chose to be tested with the ELISA test.

Her results showed a severe response to all the milks tested. These included cows' milk and sheep and goats' milk. Such a response is very unusual, and as the common factor in all these milks is the milk sugar lactose, a lactose intolerance was a real possibility.

I requested a lactose challenge test for Katy, which came back positive.

Treatment

There are two effective treatments for a patient with lactose intolerance:

1 Avoid all drinks and foods that contain milk.
2 Take milk-digesting enzymes (including lactase) before eating meals containing milk or milk products.

Katy chose to employ both treatments. She stopped using milk in most of her meals cooked at home, and took a milk-digesting enzyme formula when eating out.

Conclusion

Katy's symptoms cleared within two weeks. The improvement in Katy's symptoms, particularly her digestion of dairy products and fat, slowly began to help her lose weight. She also had more energy. Although she had not complained of feeling fatigued, she was now feeling better.

With improved digestion and food breakdown, Katy started losing about 2–3 lb (1–1^1/4 kg) each month.

At our last meeting six months after our first consultation, Katy was down to 142 lb (64 kg) which gave her a BMI of 23.5 (normal). Her own personal weight target was 132 lb (60 kg), and I could see no reason why she shouldn't achieve it.

Treating Food Intolerance

Let us assume that, with a combination of pulse testing and food avoidance, you have identified several foods that are causing or contributing to your symptoms. This is now the time to ask yourself, why? Why do common foods make you ill? More specifically for this book, why do such foods contribute to your overweight? On a more practical note, what can be done to treat such sensitivities?

When your culprit food or foods have been identified, the next obvious step is to avoid the foods. By avoiding the foods you should eventually be able to tolerate them again without a return of symptoms, when they are reintroduced into your diet. The recommended exclusion period for suspected foods is 4–8 weeks. It must be remembered that you can develop quite a severe return of symptoms if you reintroduce the foods too early and before your body has become tolerant to them.

Homoeopathic Reintroduction

I frequently prescribe a short course of homoeopathic pillules that contain the culprit foods. The amount of food actually contained in the pillules is tiny. These are taken each day for two weeks before the food itself is reintroduced into the diet.

However, even such a small amount of the food to which a patient has a proven sensitivity can provoke a rapid and severe return of symptoms. Although this occurrence is unpleasant for the patient, it serves to confirm the intolerance to that particular food.

Rotation Diet

After a period of food exclusion, culprit foods can be reintroduced on a rotation basis. This simply involves consuming the foods every 4–5 days, to allow for a progressive adjustment to them. Even with such a gradual reintroduction it is as well to keep the food portions small. So, reintroduce the foods into your eating routine slowly and carefully. If symptoms surface, you will need to avoid the food(s) again until their reintroduction does not bring on your symptoms.

Your Gut Health

If poor digestion and poor gut health have contributed to your food intolerances, it must mean that improving your digestive health and efficiency would be worthwhile. If the conditions that caused your particular food intolerance still prevail, even after diagnosis and treatment, the sensitivity may return, or you may develop symptoms from different foods.

Human Digestion

Digestion Stage by Stage

Location	Enzymes, etc.	Activity
Mouth	Ptyalin (amylase)	Digests carbohydrates
Stomach	Pepsin	Digests protein
	Mucus	Protects stomach lining
	Hydrochloric acid	Assists protein digestion
Small Intestine		
Duodenum	Pancreatic enzymes	Digests proteins
	Trypsin	Digests casein & gelatine
	Chymotrypsin	
	Steapsin	
	Amylopsin	Digests fats
	Lipase	
Liver	Bile	Assists fat digestion
Jejunum/Ileum		Absorption
Large Intestine		
(Colon)	Mucus	Elimination
Rectum	Beneficial bacteria	Elimination
Anus	Beneficial bacteria	Elimination

Treating poor digestive health falls into three chief areas: reducing environmental chemicals, normalizing digestive function, and improving your body's ability to detoxify itself.

1 Reducing Environmental Chemicals (Xenobiotics)

Xenobiotics are defined as chemicals that are foreign to the human biological system. There are many such chemicals, ranging from the obvious toxins such as alcohol, drugs, tobacco and caffeine, to toxins in our food, our water and our environment.

In excess of 3,000 chemicals are in use in the food industry, with a further 1,200 chemicals used in food packaging and preserving.

Environmental toxins including many solvents and formaldehydes, like those present in a huge range of fuels, domestic cleaners, building materials and carpets.

2 Normalizing and Improving Digestive Function

Remembering that the chief role of digestion is to break down our food or fuel into appropriate components for energy conversion, repair, defence, etc. Simply improving the efficiency of your digestive system can therefore help you to lose weight.

A normal stomach acid level or pH is essential for optimum food digestion, and to correct an inefficient digestive enzyme balance (see Chapter 7).

The Role of Fibre
The importance of fibre in human digestion has been known for many years. High-fibre diets are linked to improved digestion and bowel health, better weight control and improved circulation.

The 'Leaky Gut' Syndrome
Under normal, healthy conditions, our intestinal lining allows the components of the food we eat to be absorbed, yet protects against absorption of gut toxins. This all changes, however, if the gut's permeability is altered. The subsequent increase in the permeability adversely influences gastro-intestinal health in three ways:

1 Gut toxins and pathogens can be absorbed from the gut into the bloodstream. This can cause food intolerances, liver toxicity, immune-system deficiency and auto-immune conditions (e.g. rheumatoid arthritis).
2 The conversion of food (particularly proteins) to energy is compromised, leading to fatigue and general metabolic depression.

3   Local Irritable Bowel Syndrome-type symptoms can be caused by a leaky gut. The transit time of food is altered, giving rise to constipation and/or diarrhoea. Abdominal pain and cramping, bloating and local inflammation are all symptoms associated with the leaky gut syndrome.

3 Improving Detoxification

The liver is the chief organ responsible for detoxifying the toxins which enter our general circulation.

The liver's efficiency in detoxifying toxic compounds depends on two main factors:

1   Availability of the many nutrients that are part of the detoxifying process.
2   The type and extent of the toxic load to which the liver is exposed.

To give a clue to the complexity of this process, the long list of phytochemicals and antioxidants that are involved in detoxification includes glutathione, superoxide dismutase, catalase, vitamin E, selenium, vitamin A, N-Acetyl-Cysteine, vitamin B_2 (riboflavin), B_3 (niacin), magnesium, iron, quercetin, glycine, glutamine and methionine.

The liver is normally quite capable of dealing with toxins which develop as a result of stress, tackling infections, normal digestion and elimination. However, our total health is compromised when the liver has the additional burden of toxic exposure from a leaky gut, food allergies, gut parasites and general dysbiosis.

DYSBIOSIS
This has been defined as a condition of altered intestinal micro-ecology. The microbes, etc. involved include fungi, yeast, bacteria,

protozoa and roundworms. Stool analysis is seen as a definitive test to measure dysbiosis.

Long-term Maintenance and Treatment

Our vitality and correct body weight are influenced by many health problems not least however is our gut health and our liver efficiency. There are several areas of digestive health that we can influence ourselves, with a little care and common sense. These include:

1 Stomach acidity, emptying speed, reflux (hiatus hernia), flatulence and distention.
2 Digestive enzyme balance and efficiency.
3 Efficient food absorption and bowel health.

1 Stomach Acidity

Stomach distention with flatulence (wind) and reflux (heartburn) often occur together. Stomach acid levels and stomach-emptying speed are common causative factors.

In 1998 it was estimated that 5% of the American population suffers from dyspepsia or indigestion; of these, 40% self-medicate. We tend to associate indigestion – and many stomach symptoms – with too much stomach acid. The drugs prescribed for indigestion are often 'antacids', designed to reduce stomach acidity.

However, many stomach symptoms are more likely to be caused by a *deficiency* of stomach acid, known as *hypochlorhydria*. Such a lack of stomach acid delays digestion, causing fermentation, stomach fullness and flatulence. Protein digestion can be impaired, and the inefficient metabolism of iron, vitamin B_{12} and folic acid can lead to anaemia. Hair and nail health and low vitality are typical early symptoms of poor protein digestion.

Testing Stomach Acidity
The main test in use is not a standard NHS test. Patients attend the laboratory and swallow a small capsule that contains an exposed pH-sensing electrode. As mentioned in Chapter 5, this test is known as a gastrogram. Results obtained include the stomach acid level (pH), the pancreatic enzyme levels, and the stomach-emptying speed. With one comfortable test that lasts 45 minutes, a great deal of information is obtained. The capsule is subsequently passed and does not need to be recovered.

BICARBONATE OF SODA
A less accurate but very simple test to assess your stomach acid is as follows:

1 Dissolve a level teaspoon of bicarbonate of soda into a glass of water. (Sodium bicarbonate is an antacid prescribed to treat gastritis, gastric ulcers and acid indigestion. It is sold in most pharmacies.)
2 Drink this solution on an empty stomach.
3 As the bicarbonate is rapidly converted into gas by the action of the stomach acid, a low stomach acid level can be suspected if no belching or stomach bloating occurs within 10 minutes of drinking the solution.

2 Digestive Enzyme Balance and Efficiency

This subject will be covered more fully in Chapter 7. However, suffice to say that the most effective supplementary plant enzymes are termed 'acid-stable'. This means that they can be useful in both acid and alkaline conditions and, unlike the body's own pancreatic enzymes, they are effective when used with any stomach acid imbalance, whether the high or low acid is a result of surgery, stress, drugs or illness. These plant enzymes digest carbohydrates, fats, proteins and fibres.

Many digestive enzyme supplements also contain Betaine HCL (hydrochloric acid) to provide a boost for effective protein digestion when the stomach acidity is low.

3 Efficient Food Absorption and Bowel Health

The gut problem known as 'leaky gut syndrome' is covered earlier in this chapter. Repair of the gut and optimal bowel health depend on the following protocol:

1 Use of acid-stable digestive enzymes to normalize food digestion.
2 Identifying and repairing the gut lining, and normalizing intestinal permeability. This repair work can be done by taking supplements containing L. Glutamine, gamma-oryzanol, etc.
3 Use of antioxidants – including beta-carotene, vitamin E, zinc, selenium, ginkgo biloba and quercetin – to reduce intestinal inflammation.
4 Destroying candidiasis and other gut pathogens, and replacing them with beneficial species such as *Lactobacillus* and *Bifidobacteria*.
5 Improving the liver's health and detoxification role by eating more natural organic foods and fewer refined and processed ones, and less salt, alcohol, coffee and sugar.

Many gastro-intestinal disorders lead to a poor conversion of food to energy, nutrient deficiencies, fatigue and a general reduction in metabolic efficiency. This in turn usually causes fluid and fat retention and overweight.

Sometimes lifestyle changes may be required to normalize our digestion and achieve better health and weight. Many individuals with food intolerances achieve a normal weight when the suspect foods are identified and avoided, or when the problem is treated in some other way. Their general health and vitality are also improved.

Chapter Summary

1 Food intolerance or sensitivity is a common and often misdiagnosed cause of poor health and overweight.

2 Intolerances are frequently caused by an inefficient digestive system which can involve the digestive enzymes, stomach acidity, leaky gut and poor eating habits. Tests are available to answer questions on all these topics.

3 Food avoidance and reintroduction requires patience and discipline, but the results are usually worthwhile and weight loss is often achieved with general symptom improvement.

CHAPTER SEVEN

Food Enzymes
and Your Weight

An enzyme is a protein substance that causes chemical transformations in plants and animals. The enzyme itself is not destroyed or altered by this reaction. The enzymes in our bodies have been termed our 'labour force'. Without the action of enzymes, very little would happen to our metabolism. In fact, we would consist of a mass of inert chemicals (including proteins, vitamins, minerals and water).

When we are born, we have within us a limited enzyme supply or reserve. Unfortunately, many factors can waste our initial enzyme reserve. These include food pasteurizing, canning and microwaving. Alcohol and drugs can also serve to deplete our enzyme pool. Infections and stress may also be destructive.

The chief cause of enzyme loss or destruction, however, is cooking. Heating foods at over 130 °F/54 °C can destroy all their enzymes. As a result, we are all eating an enzyme-deficient diet.

Raw foods are enzyme-rich foods. But for those of us who do not like raw foods, fortunately there are enzyme supplements available which, taken in capsule form before food, can to a large extent compensate for the enzyme loss that occurs with cooking.

In 1930 we knew of 80 enzymes; we now know of thousands. Even so, there are many metabolic reactions occurring for which the enzymes responsible are still not known. These enzyme-requiring reactions include digestion, repair and many other functions.

Different Types of Enzymes

Enzymes can be classified into three types:

1 Metabolic enzymes – these control our metabolism.
2 Digestive enzymes – which digest our food.
3 Food enzymes – contained in food. They begin the process of digestion and assist our own digestive enzymes.

The first two types are internal (or endogenous – from within) enzymes; the third is external (or exogenous – which means 'from without').

The enzymes contained in our food are essential for the proper digestion of food. They are present in many foods, and can be taken as supplements. They work in the mouth and stomach, where they predigest our food. Plant enzymes can also work in the small intestine assisting the pancreatic enzymes to continue the digestion process.

Different kinds of digestive enzymes serve distinct functions:

Proteases	Digest proteins
Amylases	Digest carbohydrates
Lipases	Digest fats

If these enzymes are assisted by the food enzymes that occur naturally in many foods, then our enzyme reserve does not become depleted. If, however, food enzymes are largely destroyed in cooking, our own digestive enzymes must do all the work. We need more than 20 digestive enzymes, yet they are infinitely stroonger than all our other metabolic enzymes. If we are able to use the enzymes found in raw foods, our own reserve pool of metabolic enzymes will not be threatened and our own precious enzymes can be utilized to carry out their many general metabolic roles, such as health maintenance, disease prevention, body repair, etc.

Significantly cattle and sheep have a pancreas (the organ that produces many of the digestive enzymes) that is only approximately one-third the size of the human pancreas (as a percentage of total body weight) but they exist on a largely raw food diet, supplying themselves with plenty of 'external enzymes'. The use of supplemental enzymes taken with food offers a useful replacement for the food enzymes that are so frequently destroyed by cooking.

Enzymes and Your Weight

You may be thinking, but what have enzymes got to do with my weight?

As Dr Edward Howell says in his book *Enzyme Nutrition*:

> ... men in the business of extracting the maximum profit from farm animals found it was not economical to feed hogs raw potatoes. The hogs would not get fat enough. Cooking the potatoes, however, produced the fat hogs that brought the farmer the kind of money required to make a profit. This in spite of the extra expense of labour and energy involved in cooking!

In other words, raw vegetables or fruits are generally not as fattening as the same foods when cooked. Controlled trials have demonstrated that people with diabetes require less insulin if they eat raw carbohydrates compared with cooked carbohydrates. All this serves to suggest that there is a fundamental difference between raw calories and cooked calories of the same foods.

Lipase and Weight

It is not only vegetables and fruits that react in this way. Fat is also 'more fattening' when cooked than when raw. Of course, very few peoples in the world (usually only those living in isolated communities) eat raw fat. However, research into Eskimo diets in the 1920s and 1930s showed a remarkable near absence of obesity, high blood pressure and heart disease. This in spite of a high-fat, raw blubber diet. Significantly, raw fats contain the fat-digesting pancreatic enzyme lipase. This enzyme is absent in the fats cooked in the modern Western kitchen. In his landmark book *Biochemical Individuality*, Roger Williams stated that human serum lipase (lipase in the blood) shows 'at least a 30-fold range' – that is, an enormous variability exists in the human potential for fat digestion and storage. Unfortunately, very little research has been carried out to correlate human lipase levels with obesity.

There have been many raw food weight-loss diets, an example being the popular milk-and-banana diet advocated by George Harrop in the 1930s.

When I introduce patients with long-term overweight to a low-carbohydrate diet, I frequently recommend that they follow a raw fruit diet for only a day, perhaps every four or five days (for a total of around 6–8 days each month). This has the effect of 'kick-starting' their weight loss. It also serves as a valuable high-fibre detox regime, and provides useful enzymes in the raw fruits.

It is very difficult to consume more than 400–500 calories of raw food in a day. If you eat two large apples one after another, you will understand why! On page 164 I've included a copy of my fresh fruit diet, to show you the variety that's possible with this kind of method.

It has long been suspected that many obese individuals could be short of lipase. (Unfortunately, low levels of lipase are not considered to be clinically significant, as it is only high levels, as found in pancreatitis and pancreatic cancer, that are seen as important to check for.) However, in 1966 Dr David Galton tested a group of patients with an average weight of 340 lb (155 kg), and found lipase deficiency in all of them.

Age Factors

The pancreas, which supplies essential enzymes to the small intestine to assist in the digestion of proteins, carbohydrates and fats, suffers structural and functional changes with age which can reduce its enzyme output. The chief cause of this reduced flow is a narrowing or fibrosis of the main pancreatic duct. As a general rule, all our enzyme activity tends to reduce with age.

If you neglect getting enough food enzymes in your diet when you're young, your enzyme pool will diminish prematurely.

Experiments with rats have shown an enzyme tissue level difference of around 1,000 units with young rats compared with 180 units with elderly rats. (These animals were all on similar diets.)

Significantly, the thyroid gland also becomes less efficient as we grow older. In a perfect world humans would gradually lose weight with age, but the modern, denatured, cooked diet usually ensures that the opposite occurs.

Assessing Enzyme Health

Tests are available to measure your pancreatic efficiency and enzyme output. These include testing the blood levels of enzymes (e.g. amylase and lipase) or requesting a gastrogram (see Chapter 5).

Enzyme Deficiency and Overweight

The treatment of excess weight with the use of enzymes falls naturally into two stages:

1   The patient is requested to follow a diet with a high percentage of raw foods.
2   Supplementary digestive enzymes are prescribed, the dosages and variety being adjusted to individual requirements.

1 Diet

It has never been suggested by any doctors or naturopaths that a totally raw food diet is ideal for we humans. The ratio of raw to cooked foods in your diet will have to depend on many factors, including your diet's overall protein and fat content, individual taste and choice, digestive efficiency and your work output and activity levels. Although the high-protein and high-fat foods (meat, eggs, fish etc.) tend to be high in both calories and enzymes, they are usually cooked, which can reduce their enzyme content to virtually nil.

The Raw Food Diet
Many different raw food (often single- or 'mono-' food) diets have been advocated over the years, to aid a variety of health problems including obesity, fatigue, skin conditions, indigestion, gastric ulcers, asthma, hay fever, catarrh and arthritis.

It should be noted that when such diets were described as 'cures' in 17th, 18th and 19th century Europe and America, the word 'cure' referred to a course of treatment. Nowadays the word 'cure' is associated with the idea of restoration to symptom-free health – quite a different definition. These diets were designed and prescribed without any awareness or understanding of the role of food enzymes.

Many early pioneers believed that cooking food destroyed an important element in the food, which they defined as the 'life principle' or 'vital force'. They were of course describing the enzymes in food that are largely destroyed by cooking. The basis of such diets was not theoretical but practical, the patients showed symptom-relief therefore the diet was successful.

As mother-and-daughter authors Leslie and Susannah Kenton explain in their book *Raw Energy* (a well-deserved best seller), 'A mainly raw diet will help you lose weight, feel fitter and younger; it will give you a sense of super vitality and greater resistance to stress and tiredness and give relief from depression, menstrual problems and allergies.' Their book goes on to describe the many benefits of a raw food regime, including its high fibre content, inclusion of vitamin- and mineral-rich foods, and the value of nuts and seeds. The high enzyme content of raw foods, and the damage caused by cooking, are also seen as a valuable basis for the raw food approach. The authors very wisely advocate a slow transition to a 75% raw/ 25% cooked diet ratio, recommending the following strategy:

> Raw foods should be introduced into the diet slowly. Start by replacing one of your normal meals each day with a large fresh raw salad and experiment with drinking vegetable or fruit juices or herb teas instead of coffee, tea, alcohol and soft drinks.

The reader is advised to avoid processed foods, sugar-rich foods, and cows' milk products (goats' milk being preferred), and is also introduced to a guide to seed-sprouting, home-made yoghourt, and nutritious condiments and herbs. Free-range good-quality meat, game, poultry, fish and eggs are permitted (preferably conservatively cooked).

It should be remembered that enzymes are destroyed by temperatures in excess of 130 °F/54 °C. The boiling point of water is 212 °F/100 °C.

However, enzymes are not destroyed by freezing. They have been found in the flesh of mammoths who have lain under the Siberian ice for 50,000 years!

2 Supplementary Digestive Enzymes

Supplementary (exogenous) enzymes which can assist weight loss are prescribed for two reasons.

1 To generally assist the efficient digestion of fats, carbohydrates and protein foods by offering general pancreatic enzyme support.

If our food is efficiently converted to energy, there is less likelihood of fat storage. We do not need to store fat. Perhaps thousands of years ago when mankind ate 3–4 meals each week, such a mechanism provided a valuable emergency supply of fuel. With modern food distribution and refrigeration we can, and do, eat three meals each day, so individual fat storage is now quite unnecessary.

The pancreas will not become inefficient or lazy if we take supplementary enzymes, or eat lots of raw food. Pancreatic enzymes operate in the intestines, not the stomach. Food enzymes will in fact spare the pancreas from having to work harder to compensate for inadequate predigestion.

We all eat some raw foods, and primitive man certainly ate more, so it is very unlikely that the pancreatic enzymes were designed to be solely responsible for the process of digestion.

2 To specifically encourage fat digestion (by taking the fat-digesting enzyme lipase).

This enzyme serves various functions. It breaks down fat, taking stress off the liver, gall bladder and pancreas. Lipase also tends to reduce levels of LDL cholesterol (the 'bad' cholesterol) and triglycerides. Perhaps most importantly, lipase reduces excess body weight.

Lipase and Weight Loss

Bile

The chief role of bile from the gall bladder is to emulsify large fat molecules into very small molecules. This facilitates more efficient fat digestion by the lipase, and occurs in the small intestine. The lipase involved comes from the pancreas. (There is also gastric lipase, from the stomach, and hepatic lipase, from the liver.)

ANTI-OBESITY DRUGS

The anti-obesity drug Orlistat (brand name Xenical), recently available through the NHS, acts by inhibiting pancreactic lipase. It is prescribed for obese patients with a BMI in excess of 30, but side-effects include diarrhoea (with liquid, oily stools), flatulence, headaches, fatigue, anxiety and menstrual irregularities. Orlistat also compromises the absorption of the fat-soluble vitamins A, D, and E. Costing around £10 per week per patient, this drug is the pharmacological equivalent of stomach stapling.

Reducing the absorption of fat by restricting the fat-digesting enzyme lipase is not very sensible. Fat provides almost double the energy that sugar provides. It is better to encourage fat conversion to energy with increased pancreatic efficiency and an appropriate diet.

A percentage of the weight loss obtained when taking Xenical is a direct result of the very low-fat diet that is required when on the drug. All the health problems that can arise as a result of low-fat diets are exaggerated with this drug. It is a poor substitute for a thorough assessment of the causes of an individual's excess weight.

The long-term side-effects are unknown, and after the maximum 24-month treatment, patients in many cases will probably regain their surplus weight.

Lipase Deficiency

As lipase is the main enzyme prescribed for weight loss, it will pay to look more closely at its function and deficiency symptoms.

Patients with lipase deficiency generally fit into one of the following groups:

A They are fat-intolerant, experiencing nausea after eating fat, have a 'liverish' tendency with low alcohol tolerance, and often display gall-bladder symptoms. They can have a tendency to eat sugar-rich foods.

B They eat too much fat and generally prefer fat to carbohydrate foods.

Both groups tend to show high cholesterol and triglyceride blood levels, to suffer raised blood pressure and to be overweight. They often have low levels of the three fat-soluble vitamins A, D and E. These deficiencies can show themselves as poor peripheral circulation, with varicose veins, night-cramps, migraine and 'night-blindness' and dry skin.

Other common symptoms of lipase deficiency include reduced cell permeability – nutrients cannot easily enter cells, and waste materials cannot easily exit cells.

People with diabetes tend to be lipase deficient. Chronic fatigue or undiagnosed viral infections are often also a result of poor cellular activity and lipase deficiency. Muscle spasm and pain (usually spinal or intestinal), vertigo (usually with nausea and vomiting) may be linked to a low blood lipase.

N.B. A lipase deficiency is possible with as little as a 10% fall in pancreatic lipase.

Sam's Story

Consultation

Sam was the managing director of her own company. She was single, aged 37 and at least 3 stone overweight at 174 lb (79 kg) at a height of 5 ft 4 in (163 cm) and a small frame.

Her reasons for seeing me were concern over her weight and chronic indigestion. Her symptoms included stomach bloating and general discomfort after meals, coupled with, in her own words, 'a liverishness' with a very poor alcohol and fat tolerance. She felt nauseated if she ate cheese or yoghourt and, as she was obliged to eat out and socialize with clients every week, her poor food and drink tolerance were not making her life any easier.

Diet

Sam admitted to being a lazy cook, pleading lack of time. As a result she lived on microwave-cooked convenience foods. She did not eat raw food, claiming that fruit and salads invariably gave her diarrhoea.

Exercise

Sam was not interested in sport or gyms. She did, however, try to avoid overeating, and rarely ate more than 2,000 calories in a day. She also claimed to be frequently tired, but blamed her lack of vitality on her long work days and the stress of running her own business.

Diagnosis

Sam's symptoms, including her extra weight, had been with her since her early twenties. She had sought help and treatment from a variety of therapists including a medical herbalist, a nutritionist, an acupuncturist and a yoga teacher. Her doctor had, over the past two to three years, requested a battery of blood tests including thyroid function, female hormone levels and general biochemistry including the blood sugar, etc. Nothing had registered as abnormal, and so far none of the treatments prescribed had improved Sam's symptoms or reduced her weight. She had been given a diagnosis of Irritable Bowel Syndrome (IBS), had been advised to take antacids when required and to take more holidays.

Sam's intolerance of fats and alcohol – and her avoidance of all raw foods – led me to suspect that she had a pancreatic enzyme deficiency, with, more specifically, a deficiency of the fat-digesting enzyme lipase. The results of a gastrogram showed a normal gastric acid level, but delayed stomach-emptying and a decreased pancreatic enzyme function of 55% (under 70% is seen as significant). Her blood lipase level was also too low.

With little or no (external) food enzymes in her diet to support her pancreatic and metabolic (internal) enzymes, Sam's pancreas was becoming inefficient and exhausted. Instead of converting food to energy, she was converting what she ate into fat for storage. Her digestive processes were slowed down, and the delay in stomach-emptying was causing fullness and discomfort. When Sam ate the occasional raw food meal, the high-fibre content caused diarrhoea.

Treatment

I advised Sam to follow a low-carbohydrate diet and to have a side salad each day with her main meal. I knew that she was unlikely to spend hours preparing and cooking 'farmhouse' meals, but I urged her to be selective with her food buying. Good-quality organic convenience foods (including the excellent range of Linda McCartney vegetarian meals) are widely available.

I also recommended that Sam follow a raw-fruit-and-water diet one day each week, to be increased in frequency to at least two days each week. Finally, I suggested that Sam eat a single piece of fruit mid-morning and mid-afternoon on her non-fruit days.

This type of diet plan offered a low-calorie, high-fibre diet with plenty of enzyme-rich raw foods. Although the raw foods initially presented a shock to Sam's digestion, her bowels normalized within two weeks.

With her chronic weight problem in mind, I felt sure that Sam also needed to take supplementary enzymes. Her own blood lipase and reduced pancreatic enzyme activity confirmed this. I therefore prescribed two Nutri products, Similase™ and Lipase™ concentrate. (Both are described in more detail at the end of this chapter.)

Not all digestive enzyme formulas contain cellulase (for cellulose breakdown), but I felt that the Similase™ would assist Sam's ability to digest the additional fibre in her diet efficiently. These are normally taken at the onset of each meal.

The Lipase™ concentrate is taken on an empty stomach at the beginning of meals that contain fat.

Sam's intolerance of fatty foods and alcohol pointed to a degree of liver toxicity. I therefore advised her to also take a Hepa-B™ capsule each day. This is another Nutri product, and contains 200 mg each of the following plants:

- Milk thistle extract (Silymarin)
- Phyllanthus amarus
- Dandelion root

These three botanicals have been prescribed for many years to support liver health and function.

Conclusion

Over a period of four months, Sam reduced her weight by 24 lb (11 kg) to 150 lb (68 kg). This represented a weekly weight loss of 1 lb, which I considered to be satisfactory. She felt more vital, and her tolerance of fatty foods and alcohol has improved greatly. She was able to have an occasional glass of dry white wine with food without feeling queasy.

She became quite used to her 'fruit days' and regularly eats fruit only, one day a week.

I have advised Sam to continue taking a minimal maintenance dosage of the enzyme formulas and Hepa-B™. Sam's 'target' weight is 133 lb (60 kg), which she hopes to achieve in another two to three months. With her present diet and enzyme support, she should be able to achieve and maintain such a weight.

Enzyme Treatment

As I have described earlier in this chapter, natural plant enzymes can be prescribed to supplement our own digestive enzymes. The enzymes that our digestive system produces are boosted by the enzymes that naturally occur in raw foods. It is the reduction of food enzymes by modern processing and cooking that justifies the use of supplementary enzymes.

Supplementary enzymes can be used either for general support or for a specific health problem such as lactose intolerance.

The majority of concentrated enzyme supplements are derived from plants (such as papaya and pineapple), and they can be safely prescribed for a variety of ailments. However, in common with many nutritional supplements, the selection and dosage requirements for specific health problems may require the help of a qualified health practitioner or naturopath.

Enzymes to Combat Overweight

The main enzyme for fat digestion is lipase (already described earlier in this chapter). The chief supplement I find of value when I suspect a lipase deficiency is called Lipase™ concentrate (Nutri). It is a very concentrated plant-based enzyme that is active and stable in acid and alkaline conditions and provides assistance for fat digestion.

Taking a 'broad spectrum' enzyme complex with other nutrients regularly could help many individuals to process food more efficiently. In mid-life and old age, many of us have reduced our enzyme reserve, and supplementary enzymes will assist our conversion of food to energy rather than to fat stores. Our enzyme potential can thus also be directed towards other metabolic activities aside from digestion.

In his book *Enzyme Nutrition*, Dr Edward Howell describes the enzyme deficit of age as follows:

> It can be accepted as a working rule that the enzyme potential is limited and withers as time marches on. The more lavishly a young body gives up its enzymes, the sooner the state of enzyme poverty, or old age, is reached.

I shall now describe the four general-purpose enzyme formulae that I prescribe to improve digestive efficiency, energy and weight control. The ingredient lists indicate their versatility and clinical value.

Enzyme Formula	Description	Ingredients
Similase™ (Nutri)	A highly concentrated and gentle plant enzyme digestive formula, stable and active in a wide pH range (pH 2–12), from the acid environment of the stomach to the alkaline environment of the small intestine. Derived from natural plant sources, this formula is well tolerated and provides balanced assistance for the digestion of protein, fat and carbohydrates. (Not recommended for individuals with gastritis or ulcers.)	Protease, amylase, cellulose, lipase, phytase, lactase, sucrase and maltase

Gastric Complex™ (Nutri)	A soothing digestive formula which combines highly concentrated plant enzymes (active in a wide pH range) with gamma oryzanol (from rice bran oil) and other botanicals. Due to its gentle action, this formula reduces stress on the gastrointestinal system and is well tolerated by those with a sensitive gastrointestinal tract.	Marshmallow root, slippery elm bark, gamma oryzanol (from rice bran oil), amylase, lipase and cellulase
Fibre Formula™ (Nutri)	A special blend of soothing herbs, probiotics and plant enzymes, combined in a high-fibre formula designed for optimal bowel function and toxin removal. Helps to maintain the muscle tone of the colonic walls, and to support normal function of the bowels.	Psyllium hull powder, oat bran powder, bentonite powder, guar gum, marshmallow root, prune powder, vitamin C, bromelain, papain, ginger root, echinacea, goldenseal root, cranesbill

| Hypo-D™ (Nutri) | Hypo-D is a potent combination of hydrochloric acid, digestive enzymes and ox bile – the First Phase operates in the stomach, the Second Phase in the duodenum. | First Phase: Betaine HCL, L-Glutamine acid HCL, pepsin, papain Second Phase: Pancreatin, pancrealipase, amylase, bromelain, ox bile and parotid |

Enzymes for Specific Health Problems

In addition to combating overweight, enzyme formulae are available to treat the following health problems:

constipation
hypochlorhydria (low stomach acid)
food intolerances
gluten intolerance
lactose intolerance
candidiasis
short-chain fatty acid deficiency
dysbiosis
toxic bowel
leaky gut syndrome
intestinal wind and bloating
IBS
blood sugar control

Chapter Summary

1 Enzyme imbalance or deficiency can cause poor digestion and weight gain.
2 Enzymes are required to digest our food, but many other enzymes are needed to control the chemistry of our metabolism.
3 Although we manufacture and release our own enzymes, they are also included in raw foods (but destroyed by heating and cooking).
4 Enzyme supplements, extracted from plants, can offer general digestive support or make up for specific deficiencies.
5 Our enzyme reserve declines with age, and all the more quickly with a diet that includes only cooked foods.
6 General or specific enzyme supplements can improve digestive efficiency, alleviate or cure food intolerances, and help you to lose excess weight.

Fresh Fruit Low-calorie Diet

Every four to five days, eat only from the fruits listed below. Do not have any one type of fruit more than three times daily, and avoid fruit that you suspect you may be allergic to (for example, strawberries and oranges).

Have up to a maximum of NINE pieces of fruit daily, preferably at normal meal times.

Use only fresh ripe fruit (or frozen soft fruit), and avoid unnecessary shredding, chopping and peeling.

Do NOT add sugar or artificial sweeteners.

Drink only bottled mineral water, as much as desired.

Calorie count: approximately 350–500 calories depending on selection. (Figures apply to whole fresh fruit unless otherwise stated.)

Apple (medium)	50 calories
Apricots (5)	30 calories
Blackberries (4 oz)	35 calories
Blackcurrants (4 oz)	35 calories
Cherries (4 oz)	48 calories
Grapefruit (medium)	35 calories
Figs (fresh green, 4 oz)	48 calories
Grapes (12)	50 calories
Lychees (4)	32 calories
Melon (8 oz)	30 calories
Orange (medium)	45 calories
Peach	35 calories
Pear (medium)	45 calories
Pineapple (4 oz)	52 calories
Plums (3 medium)	35 calories
Pomegranate	65 calories
Raspberries (4 oz)	30 calories
Redcurrants (4 oz)	30 calories
Strawberries (4 oz)	30 calories
Tangerine/Mandarin	20 calories
Watermelon (8 oz)	24 calories

CHAPTER EIGHT

Hormones and Your Weight

From puberty to old age, a woman's hormones exert a profound influence on her mental and physical health. There is a large catalogue of disorders, uniquely female and hormone-linked, which invariably include weight gain as one of their symptoms.

Excessive weight is not always caused by particular ailments, however. In addition to disorders or illnesses – examples being PMS, hypothyroidism (underactive thyroid) PCOS (Polycystic Ovary Syndrome, see page 177), many women become overweight at puberty, during pregnancy or simply as a result of lifestyle problems or the ageing process. This type of weight gain can be a chronically slow process over 10 or 20 years, and resulting from a simple hormone imbalance or deficiency. A subtle change in a woman's food intake–energy output ratio can also lead to gradual weight gain. There is evidence to suggest that simply following the wrong diet for your metabolic type can result in increased weight.

Puberty

With the onset of menstruation, usually around the age of 12–14, the female metabolism can become imbalanced. Many patients who consult me with stubborn overweight declare that their symptoms began in their early teenage years.

The cells in the ovaries secrete the female hormones which help girls develop into women. Part of this transition leads to a laying down of fat in the hips, thighs and breasts.

All this is an essential part of the maturing process. If, however, there is an imbalance in the hormones, and a girl passes through puberty with an excessive weight load, a pattern may be set for adult obesity.

A combination of female hormone imbalance, lack of exercise and the modern tendency to snack on high-starch foods has resulted in 20% of children in the US being seriously overweight. For girls in the UK between the ages of 4 and 12, this figure is 15%.

Oestrogen

Many female health problems, including weight gain, are caused by oestrogen replacement or oestrogen excess. The American nutritionist Carlton Fredericks has written that 'It is a paradox that oestrogen is routinely used to treat conditions caused by oestrogen.' Excessive oestrogen leads to oestrogen dominance.

Dr John Lee, who defined the term 'Oestrogen Dominance', maintains that excessive oestrogen can cause weight gain as a result of two changes: fluid retention and the accumulation of extra fatty tissue around the hips and thighs. Any extra fluid retained can lead to salt cravings, just exacerbating the problem.

Small wonder that so many women complain of weight gain when taking the contraceptive pill or HRT. The long-term side-effects of the 'morning after' pill have yet to be recognized. Significantly, it is likely that young teenagers will now have access to a new 'Pill', with an oestrogen content around 50 times that of the traditional contraceptive pill.

The Role of the Liver

Oestrogen excess is normally controlled by the liver. One of its many functions is to break oestrogen down into the harmless hormone oestriole, which is then eliminated in the urine. Poor liver health can compromise the efficiency of this process, and too much alcohol, caffeine and sugar can all lower the liver's vitality. Other requirements include the availability of various members of the vitamin B family, and adequate protein in your diet. Many nutritionists prescribe high-protein, low-carbohydrate diets, alongside vitamin B complex supplements, to reduce oestrogen dominance and activity.

Oestrogen and Progesterone

We often read that oestrogen should be prescribed with progesterone, to achieve a natural and appropriate balance. Unlike oestrogen, progesterone acts as a natural diuretic (fluid-reducer), burning fat for energy and lowering the body's total cholesterol.

Unfortunately the average diet in the UK and the US is low in vitamin B_6 (pyridoxine). This vitamin is the most valuable and effective nutrient to assist progesterone production and oestrogen control. This explains its unique value in reducing the symptoms of PMS (pre-menstrual syndrome).

Problems Caused by Excess Oestrogen

In addition to fat and fluid increase, excessive oestrogen can also contribute to PMS, mood changes and sugar cravings. On a more serious level, breast cancer, blood-clotting, uterine fibroids, PCOS and endometriosis are also linked to elevated oestrogen activity.

When women are prescribed oestrogen as a hormone replacement following the menopause or a hysterectomy, no one stops to ask why neither young girls before puberty, nor men, suffer flushes and other symptoms as a result of their low oestrogen levels.

Satisfactory hormone replacement and subsequent balancing can often be achieved with nutritional support of the liver, coupled with appropriate non-hormonal supplements.

PMS (Pre-menstrual Syndrome)

Many women who suffer from PMS experience a weight increase of up to 6–7 lb before each period. As most of this increase is a direct result of fluid retention, their weight usually returns to normal when the period is over.

However, the return to normal weight does not always occur. Many patients report to me that their weight increase, with puffy ankles and legs, has developed into a permanent feature, this extra weight increasing more and more with their PMS each month.

The exact cause of PMS has remained a controversial subject for many years, the debate being polarized into two main areas: hormonal causes, and nutritional causes.

Hormonal Causes

Either a raised oestrogen level (the contraceptive pill can trigger or worsen PMS) or a reduced progesterone level have been identified as common causes. Even a subtle shift in the ratio of these two hormones can contribute to PMS symptoms.

The ovaries produce progesterone at the mid-cycle ovulation. It therefore follows that, as progesterone chiefly influences the second half of the cycle, at the time when PMS symptoms develop, a low level of progesterone may be a common cause of PMS.

I frequently prescribe a 2–3 month trial on soya-based natural progesterone cream.

NATURAL PROGESTERONE CREAM

This cream, known as Serenity for Women™, is a 'hypo-allergenic premium quality natural moisturizing cream free from all common allergens, containing Pharmaceutical Grade unadulterated natural progesterone, extracted from the soy plant'. The cream also contains aloe vera, yam extract, black cohosh, Siberian ginseng, complex grain oil and vitamin E. The progesterone content (2.1%) has been calculated to provide progesterone in appropriate amounts to balance unopposed oestrogen (oestrogen dominance). A 2-oz (57-gm/60-ml) jar contains not less than 1,260 mg of natural progesterone.

YAM EXTRACT CREAMS

These creams do not guarantee a natural progesterone content. However, the yam extract is thought to convert into progesterone. Many of the yam-based creams also contain plant extracts of black cohosh, damiana, agnus castus and dong quai, which may be responsible for the beneficial effects.

A trial use of progesterone cream offers a safe and effective method to assess the need for progesterone, which is confirmed by subsequent symptom-relief.

Low-Level Progesterone and Hypothyroidism

The symptoms caused by a low level of progesterone are very similar to the symptoms of an underactive thyroid. As a result, a misdiagnosis can often occur.

Dr John R. Lee, who is known for his work on oestrogen dominance, has stated that a low progesterone level is often misdiagnosed as a thyroid deficiency. The symptoms that can develop include:

- Weight increase
- Fluid retention
- Joint and muscle pain
- Poor circulation
- Reduced sex drive

- Headaches
- Depression
- Low blood sugar
- Potassium-sodium imbalance
- Zinc and copper reductions

Readers will see similarities with the symptoms of hypothyroidism (see Chapter 9).

Reduced thyroid function can also, in my opinion, cause PMS. As long ago as 1888 the Clinical Society of London published a report which showed that 35% of women with hypothyroidism had menstrual symptoms. The benefits of thyroid therapy for a variety of menstrual disorders including PMS have been confirmed and demonstrated over many years. (See Chapter 9 for more about the thyroid.)

Other Hormonal Causes
Reduced levels of the adrenal hormone DHEA (dehydro-epi-androsterone) have also been implicated as a cause of PMS.

Patients with PCOS (Polycystic Ovary Syndrome – see page 177) and endometriosis frequently suffer from PMS. Subsequent improvement in these two conditions tends to reduce their PMS symptoms.

Nutritional Causes

Many doctors and naturopaths point to poor nutrition as a key cause of PMS. Low levels of the B vitamins, particularly B_6, vitamin D and magnesium, when coupled with a low-fat and low-protein, high-sugar diet, have all been seen to cause or worsen PMS. A deficiency of the essential fatty acids (Omega 3 and 6) have also been known to be causative factors. Hence the huge interest in the use of Evening Primrose Oil (Omega 6) for the treatment of PMS.

What is termed the 'leaky gut syndrome', or altered gut permeability, with associated systemic candidiasis, has also been associated with PMS.

I have found that, in common with many other health problems, PMS is frequently the result of several causes. However, it is often possible to relieve the symptoms of PMS and at the same time achieve a substantial weight reduction. A comprehensive cause assessment, followed by the appropriate treatment, is essential.

Perimenopause

The concept of early menopause, with women experiencing symptoms as young as 35, is relatively new. The symptoms can include irregular bleeding with missed periods, fluid retention, low blood sugar, depressed thyroid activity, fatigue and weight gain. These symptoms occur largely as a direct result of 'unopposed' oestrogen (high oestrogen with low progesterone).

When ovulation does not take place, progesterone is not produced but a regular and constant oestrogen level is maintained, resulting in a missed period. If a woman does not bleed for 2–3 months, only the oestrogen level will rise, as it is unopposed by the progesterone control effect.

Many women discover that as they enter their late thirties they experience missed periods coupled with gradual weight gain. There may well be other reasons for such weight gain, but if a woman experiences missed periods plus the other symptoms linked to perimenopause, a hormonal cause can be suspected.

Hysterectomy and Weight

Hysterectomy remains a controversial procedure. Around 800,000 of these 'overnight menopause' operations are performed each year in the US, and 50% of the American female population will have a hysterectomy some time in their lives. (These figures compare with 10% of the Scandinavian female population.)

Although modern anaesthetics and after-care renders surgery more comfortable and safe compared with past centuries, a hysterectomy is still a great shock to the female metabolism. The main after-effect of such surgery is weight increase. Many women complain of a ballooning of their weight following their hysterectomy, while others suffer a delayed weight increase which occurs 18–24 months after surgery. (Possibly a result of the ovaries finally shutting down.)

There is little doubt that many women put on weight following hysterectomy. This operation has been likened to an 'overnight' menopause, and the menopause can adversely influence female health in many ways:

- Reduction in oestrogen
- Increase in body fat
- Increased risk of heart disease, osteoporosis (brittle bones), and breast cancer.

I have talked to patients who have suffered a weight increase of 30–40 lb (13–18 kg) following hysterectomy, yet they have assured me that their activities and diet have not changed since their operation.

The oft-stated medical opinion that women have no use for their ovaries after a certain age is simply not correct. The hormone testosterone, which fuels a woman's libido, is produced by the ovaries. Removal of the ovaries also causes a woman to lose the chief source of female hormones (progesterone and oestrogen).

It is difficult to justify removal of the ovaries as routine. For many women a partial hysterectomy, which involves uterine removal only, leads to fewer symptoms post-operatively, although the shock of surgery can render the ovaries useless after 18–24 months.

Oestrogen and progesterone need to work together in harmony. Following hysterectomy, some oestrogen is still available, being produced by the adrenal glands and tissue fat reserves, but progesterone production virtually ceases. Such a deficiency can adversely influence the adrenal stress hormones, leading to the development of stress-related disorders (anxiety, depression, etc.). This suggests that any hormone replacement therapy (HRT) after a hysterectomy needs to consist chiefly of progesterone.

Jane's Story

Consultation

Jane was aged 48 when she consulted me with overweight, depression and anxiety. Prior to her hysterectomy five years earlier, she had weighed 142 lb (65 kg) which, at a height of 5 ft 6 in (168 cm), gave her a BMI of 23 (normal).

Jane began to gain weight 3–4 weeks after the hysterectomy, even with the help of HRT, prescribed by her doctor shortly after the operation. A year after the surgery she weighed almost 168 lb (76 kg).

Although a self-confessed 'anxious worrier', Jane had managed to stop her smoking habit of 20 cigarettes daily two years previously, and within a short time had gained another 15 lb (7 kg), so that by the time she consulted me she weighed 186 lb (84 kg), with a BMI of 30 (just into the 'obese' range).

As far as Jane was concerned, the changes to her body as a result of her hysterectomy had caused her rapid weight increase.

It became obvious to me that Jane could be suffering symptoms of progesterone deficit and resulting oestrogen dominance. It is important to have an optimal balance between oestrogen and progesterone. After a hysterectomy, a woman's body can still produce oestrogen from fatty tissues and adrenal activity. Progesterone is also a biological precursor for the production of oestrogen – in other words, progesterone can convert to oestrogen, but not the other way around.

Treatment

Jane's treatment was triple-pronged: we addressed her diet, need for supplements, and exercise levels.

DIET

Being an ex-smoker, Jane still retained a strong sugar craving, with a tendency to low blood sugar or, as she described it, 'shakes and yawnings' usually occurring on waking and if meals were delayed for any reason. I therefore advised her to follow a low-carbohydrate and frequent, small-meal (5–6 meals daily) eating plan. This sounds like a great deal of food, however the 'meals' are in reality snacks and the total calorie count is around 1,800 calories per day.

SUPPLEMENTS

I prescribed a plant-based natural progesterone cream for Jane. This formula also contains the herbs to assist female hormone regulation: agnus castus, damiana, dong quai and black cohosh.

Agnus castus is a particularly valuable remedy for low progesterone symptoms. It opposes excessive oestrogen, assists fluid retention, and alleviates nervous tension and depression. It also stimulates the production of progesterone and reduces the production of oestrogen.

EXERCISE

Jane's overweight and resulting lethargy had caused her to reduce any exercise to a minimum. I advised her to allow time for a brisk walk each day, and to swim at least twice weekly.

Conclusion

Jane needed to lose 45 lb (21 kg). After four months on her new regime of frequent small meals, exercise and progesterone cream, she had lost 18 lb (8 kg), giving her a BMI of 28. After six months she was down to 154 lb (70 kg) with a BMI of just under 26. I was confident that with a further 2–3 months on the programme Jane would achieve her target of 140 lb (64 kg), and a return to her original BMI of 23–24.

Although it is tempting to seek a single cause of excessive weight, Jane's case demonstrates that very often several causes co-exist. There can be a dominant cause (in Jane's case the oestrogen-progesterone imbalance), yet secondary factors may also need to be addressed, including diet and exercise levels.

The Menopause and Weight

The menopause can be defined as an oestrogen deficit causing cessation of periods. The average age for the onset of the menopause is 51, although there is a wide age range, from 45 to 60. Many women find they go through the menopause at the same age as their mothers did.

While most women pass through this time with a minimum of symptoms, others however suffer mood changes, fatigue, insomnia, joint and muscle pain and stiffness and headaches. As I have written earlier, many women gain weight during and after the menopause.

After periods have stopped for 12 months, it is assumed that the menopause is completed.

When the ovaries start to fail with the coming of the menopause, a pituitary compensation is triggered and the pituitary hormone FSH (Follicle Stimulating Hormone) stimulates the continued functioning of the ovaries. This hormone, which is termed a gonadotropin is the chief cause of the hot flushes or 'flashes' that usually occur during and after the menopause.

The menopause should not be seen as an illness but a normal part of life. The transition from a normal monthly cycle to the ovaries 'shutting down' should be smooth and symptom-free. Nutritional treatment offers hope for this and for weight gain to be reduced, along with general symptom improvement.

PCOS (Polycystic Ovary Syndrome)

The symptoms of PCOS include overweight, increased facial hair, acne, infertility, irregular periods, chronic fatigue, mood swings, joint and muscle pain, hair loss, depression and poor libido. Any two or three of these symptoms would knock a woman's self-esteem, but to suffer the full set (as many PCOS sufferers do), can inspire real depression and despair.

What is PCOS?

The diversity of symptoms, coupled with the fact that all the symptoms can have other causes, has lead to PCOS being virtually ignored as a health problem. It is only over the last two years that magazine articles and books are being written about this condition, and public awareness is increasing.

Although 'discovered' in the 1930s, the syndrome was thought only to include obesity, amenorrhoea (lack of periods) and excessive facial and body hair. I became interested in PCOS for two principal reasons: It can cause obesity, and it is associated with a condition known as insulin resistance or Syndrome X.

Causes of PCOS

PCOS is essentially an ovarian hormone imbalance. This causes an exaggerated pituitary response, which leads to excessive LH (Leutinizing Hormone) and FSH (Follicle Stimulating Hormone) levels, which interfere with testosterone and, ultimately, oestrogen production.

Luteinizing Hormone (LH)

LH influences the second half of the female cycle and stimulates the ovaries to produce testosterone, which in a normal cycle is then converted to oestrogen. The elevation of LH provides one explanation for the raised testosterone levels, the hirsuitism and acne so common in PCOS. Whether this is a cause or an effect is subject to some dispute and ongoing research.

The Insulin Link

Many women with PCOS have raised levels of blood insulin (see Chapter 2). This is termed *hyperinsulinism* or – when the raised levels are a direct result of compensation for a poor insulin effect on the blood sugar – *insulin resistance*.

The link between PCOS and insulin resistance was identified around 20 years ago. Research confirmed that insulin tends to stimulate ovarian production of the androgen testosterone – and an excess of free or unbound testosterone causes many of the symptoms of PCOS.

The connection between overweight PCOS patients and their testosterone levels is that, as with LH, insulin stimulates an increase in their ovarian manufacture of testosterone. Some 75% of overweight women with PCOS show raised insulin levels – clearly a major factor in causing raised testosterone levels.

Insulin resistance can also cause a tendency to low blood sugar (hypoglycaemia), which can in turn lead to sugar craving and overweight.

In his excellent book *Genetic Nutritioneering*, Jeffrey Bland identifies the following characteristics of insulin resistance:

1 Tendency to gain fat in the upper body
2 Menstrual irregularities and PCOS in women
3 Marginally elevated LDL ('bad') cholesterol
4 Marginally elevated blood fats (triglycerides)
5 Marginally elevated blood pressure
6 A sweet tooth
7 Symptoms that resemble hypoglycaemia
8 A family history of maturity-onset diabetes.

The concept of producing too much insulin may seem strange to many readers, probably because insulin is usually discussed within the context of a deficiency, as in the case of diabetes.

Insulin resistance defines a condition where more insulin than normal is needed to maintain optimal levels of blood sugar. In other words, the pancreas revs up and a higher level of circulating insulin is established. If this continues the pancreas can become exhausted, eventually leading to diabetes. Unfortunately, the high carbohydrate Western diet can cause overproduction of insulin, increased fat storage, and many other health problems.

Insulin – A Brief History
Many hundreds and thousands of years ago, humans did not have access to supermarkets, farms did not exist and food preservation methods were unknown. Food was obtained by hunting and gathering, and like many present-day carnivores in the animal kingdom, humans were probably lucky to eat a full meal once or twice each week. This feast-or-famine pattern led their bodies to overproduce insulin.

One of the chief roles of insulin is to facilitate food storage. Carbohydrates are converted to glycogen and lodged in the liver and muscle, while fats are stored as triglycerides. If these stores could not be utilized, the food would simply be converted into energy for muscle use and other metabolic requirements. Therefore, insulin resistance allowed our ancestors to store the fat they needed for times when no food was available.

Unfortunately there is no evidence to suggest that this system has adapted to the 21st-century food intake. Instead of eating a full meal perhaps once or twice weekly, as our ancestors did, we now tend to eat three times each day. Fat storage is therefore no longer necessary. This means that, for those who have a tendency to insulin resistance (which can be identified and measured), weight loss on a typical Western diet is virtually impossible. The high carbohydrate content of our diets, including refined starches and sugar, leads to the yo-yo effect of high blood sugar followed by low blood sugar, caused by an excessive insulin response. The low blood sugar causes a heightened appetite (especially for sugar-rich foods) and a vicious circle is established.

Elaine's Story

Elaine had been given a diagnosis of Polycystic Ovary Syndrome (PCOS) by her doctor two years previously. This diagnosis was based on a positive ultrasound scan coupled with a raised blood testosterone and mildly raised total cholesterol and triglyceride levels.

Consultation

Elaine was aged 32 years and suffered a vast array of symptoms. These included:

Hair	Elaine had suffered excessive facial and body hair since puberty.
Acne	For over 18 years this unsightly condition was over her face, chest and upper back. Other skin symptoms included poor healing and frequent unexplained bruising, and extreme sensitivity to sunlight.
Fatigue and depression	So often these two symptoms occur together. Elaine had suffered severe fatigue and depression since her late teens.
Overweight	Although quite tall, at 5 ft 11 in (180 cm), Elaine was still too heavy for her height, being 192 lb (87 kg) – giving her a BMI of 26.6. She had two children, aged 4 and 2, and she had been overweight since halfway through her first pregnancy.

Digestion	Elaine claimed to 'react' to foods, with stomach fullness and chronic constipation. She chiefly blamed dairy foods and bread.
Circulation	Elaine felt cold all the time, with frequent paraesthesia (pins and needles) in the hands, varicose veins, haemorrhoids and night cramp.
General Symptoms	Her libido was non-existent, her mood was unpredictable and her powers of concentration and short-term memory were both very poor. She complained of stiffness and aching in the ankles and knees. Her periods were erratic, and she suffered from PMS involving four to five days premenstrually when she would experience serious sugar cravings.

Diagnosis

Although I was tempted to regard Elaine's many symptoms as being a result of PCOS, I thought it wise to consider other possible causes. As I have written elsewhere in this book, many people suffer several parallel health problems, and as each condition can throw up its own symptom-picture, diagnosis is never easy.

Elaine's doctor had diagnosed PCOS (although no treatment had been offered). It is known that ovarian cysts can appear even on the scans of symptom-free patients. It is also accepted that elevation of the male hormone testosterone is the most common diagnostic feature of PCOS.

Tests

I requested a set of tests for Elaine in an attempt to identify the cause or causes of her many symptoms. These tests confirmed that Elaine's

Luteinizing Hormone level was raised, as was her insulin. Her total cholesterol, LDL cholesterol and triglycerides were also above the range of reference. She had a normal red and white cell count, no anaemia, and her glucose and other tests were all normal. Her thyroid test results were also well within the normal ranges. A serum mineral profile, however, showed low levels of zinc, magnesium and chromium.

Treatment

As excess weight is closely linked with hyperinsulinism, and the excess insulin will increase levels of testosterone in the body, readers will not be surprised to read that the symptoms of those who suffer from PCOS get worse as their weight increases. Conversely, even a 5% or 10% reduction in body weight can dramatically improve the symptoms of PCOS. (This means that if a woman weighing 168 lb/76 kg can manage to lose 8–16 lb/4–7 kg, she can feel a great deal better.)

I placed Elaine on a low carbohydrate diet to assist the insulin resistance, and prescribed the following remedies and supplements.

Agnus Castus (Chaste Tree)

This plant remedy stimulates production of progesterone and reduces oestrogen. It acts as a general female hormone regulator and assists such conditions as PMS, fluid retention and depression.

GTF Complex™

This complex was formulated by me for Nutri Ltd to provide all the nutrients to enable the body to utilize glucose effectively as a fuel. Primarily designed to treat hypoglycaemia (low blood sugar), it is also prescribed for insulin resistance. It contains zinc, chromium and magnesium – the three minerals that were deficient in Elaine's serum mineral profile test. The complete constituents of GTF Complex™ are described in Chapter 2.

Carnitine

This valuable amino-acid (protein) helps our metabolism to transport and burn fats for weight loss. Dr Atkins states in his book *Dr Atkins Vita-Nutrient Solution* that 'The release of fat for use as fuel makes this nutrient an important adjunct to any weight-loss or exercise efforts.'

Carnitine is chiefly found in red meat, and is not found in vegetable protein. (This suggests that vegetarians, vegan and those on low-protein diets may be at risk of carnitine deficiency.) A deficiency tends to increase our cholesterol and triglyceride levels. Significantly, carnitine has great value in improving blood flow to the hands and feet. Elaine, you may recall, suffered cramp, coldness and paraesthesia to the extremities.

Acety-L-Carnitine (ALC)

This can be defined as a 'super' carnitine. Unfortunately it is not readily available from health food suppliers.

Conclusion

After six months of treatment Elaine had lost a total of 16 lb (7 kg), with a BMI reduced from 26.6 to 24.4 – which took her into the upper end of the 'normal' range. Of all her symptoms, her skin had improved most dramatically, and her energy levels, joint and muscle symptoms were considerably improved.

Rechecks on her blood showed a gradual improvement in the levels of insulin, LH and lipids (fats), although there was clearly more work to do. Her circulation had improved and the weight loss and change of diet had reduced her digestive symptoms.

PCOS is a complex problem, and I feel sure that the most satisfactory approach is to improve the vitality by glucose-insulin balancing and to reduce the body fats in the tissues and blood.

Elaine will probably need further treatment guidance for another 6–9 months, but progress and weight loss are being achieved.

Chapter Summary

1 Throughout a woman's life, almost any imbalance in her hormones results in unwanted weight.

2 Hormones can influence the metabolic rate (hypothyroidism), the blood sugar levels (PCOS), fluid control (PMS), fat metabolism (menopause) and many other areas.

3 So often a female hormone disorder (e.g. an oestrogen–progesterone imbalance) requires a gentle whole-body approach using nutrition and safe plant supplements in place of prescription hormones and drugs.

4 Puberty, menstruation, pregnancy and the menopause should not be excuses for symptoms. If symptoms do surface at these times in a woman's life, there are always reasons that need to be identified and treated, such as PMS, postnatal depression, pregnancy sickness and post-menopausal flushings.

5 Hormonal overweight can be successfully treated in many cases by diagnosing and treating the causes, and not only the symptoms.

CHAPTER NINE

The Thyroid Gland and Your Weight

The thyroid is a small gland weighing between 8 and 40 gm (approximately $1/4$–$1^1/2$ oz) situated in the front of the neck. It controls our metabolism in various ways.

Underactive Thyroid – The Symptoms

An underactive thyroid gland (hypothyroidism – known as *myxoedema* when severe) can give rise to a host of symptoms including fatigue, hair loss, depression, muscle and joint pain and, significantly for this book, weight gain.

A diagnosis of hypothyroidism is dependent on blood test results. If the patient's thyroid hormones are below the 'normal range', hypothyroidism is diagnosed. This is then usually followed up with a prescription for the thyroid hormone thyroxine.

I regularly see patients who are suffering many typical symptoms of hypothyroidism, yet who have been reassured that their thyroid results are with the 'normal range' and therefore that the thyroid does not require treatment. Such patients are defined as 'clinically hypothyroid' (presenting symptoms of a depressed thyroid) but 'biochemically euthyroid' (having a normal thyroid according to the interpretation of blood test results).

This diagnostic paradox leads to a situation where many exhausted, overweight patients who are suffering borderline hypothyroidism are told to eat less, and are frequently offered a prescription for anti-depressants.

Diagnosing Hypothyroidism

The criterion for thyroid diagnosis in the UK does not always include the clinical assessment of a patient's symptoms, priority being given to the blood test findings. The result of this is that mild ('sub-clinical') conditions are not diagnosed and treated. Yet with the known variability in the size of the human thyroid, it seems to me that symptom-assessment should always be an essential component of diagnosis.

Prior to the 1940s, blood thyroid hormone measurements were not available, and only a patient's symptoms determined the diagnosis. In addition, the 'normal ranges' defined by hospital laboratories show considerable variations throughout the country. The prescription for the thyroid hormone thyroxine (or T4) is currently free in the UK, but thyroxine is only prescribed if the patient is below the lower end of 'normal range'. This means that symptom severity is discounted or ignored in favour of a rigid compliance with 'normal ranges'.

To compound this situation, the 'normal ranges' in the UK are becoming lower each year. In many European countries, the ranges for thyroxine are between 12 or 13 and 28. The UK figures vary from 7.5–21 up to 10–25. You will see from these variations that a fatigued, overweight patient with a blood thyroxine of say, 12.5, would be sent away without treatment in the UK but diagnosed as hypothyroid in France or Germany. I have never seen reference ranges for thyroid hormones lower than UK ranges.

This rather rigid, laboratory-based approach to diagnosis seems to me to be very unfair to the patient. There are symptom severity variations in practically all health problems. A good example is diabetes. A patient with mild diabetes may only be required to alter his or her diet to achieve a stable blood sugar target. However, a person with insulin-dependent diabetes may require 5–6 insulin injections daily just to stay alive.

The majority of overweight patients who visit me have been diagnosed as euthyroid (normal thyroid). However, the clinical evidence, symptom picture and the correct interpretation of test results frequently confirm that their thyroid is in fact under-functioning.

Meg's Story

I have seen many overweight patients similar to Meg. However, I have chosen to describe her case in this chapter because her health history illustrates so well the complexity of the causes and effects of hypothyroidism and overweight. Meg's case also demonstrates the variations that exist in hypothyroid diagnosis and treatment.

Consultation

When Meg first consulted me she was aged 57, 5 ft 7 in (170 cm) tall and weighed 210 lb (95 kg) – giving her a BMI of 34. She described a very long list of symptoms in addition to her overweight. These included fatigue, poor short-term memory, poor concentration, cold hands and feet, headaches, neck and shoulder pain, low back stiffness, night cramps, constipation, high blood pressure, raised cholesterol, depression and mood swings. Many of her symptoms were worse on rising, and improved towards the end of the day.

Symptoms

When patients like Meg present 15–20 symptoms, it is very tempting for practitioners to define them as psychosomatic cases and to prescribe anti-depressants. (Indeed, many of my hypothyroid patients have been offered anti-depressants.) The opinion of many doctors is that clinical depression can itself cause a galaxy of symptoms including fatigue, joint and muscle pain and stiffness, insomnia, headaches, etc. However, when a patient's thyroid is depressed, they *will* become mentally and physically depressed. Their depression is a symptom, not the underlying cause of their health problems. Significantly, many American psychiatrists and doctors are now prescribing low-dosage thyroxine for their depressed patients, based on the reasoning that depressed patients are usually also physically depressed (fatigued). So they treat the metabolism with thyroid support, to improve patients' energy and subsequently reduce their mental depression. Low-dose thyroxine (e.g. 25 mcg) does not lead to a dependency and can be discontinued after symptom-relief has been achieved. (See References – *The Thyroid Solution*.)

Examination and History

In spite of her symptoms, Meg was a full-time junior school teacher and was married with four children.

Although she had never suffered any major health problems, she had experienced a great deal of stress over the previous 30 years:

Age 22	Birth of son, cot death aged 3 months
23	Birth of second son, caesarean section
32	Divorce. Thyroid enlargement (goitre) and weight down to 114 lb (51 kg)
38	Remarriage after being a single parent for six years. Three young step-children
42	Total hysterectomy; weight at 133 lb (60 kg)
44	Weight ballooned to 175 lb (79 kg) 18 months after the operation.

By the time she was 48 Meg weighed 192 lb (87 kg) – and an explanation was found for her overweight and other symptoms. Blood tests confirmed that she was suffering from hypothyroidism.

When Meg consulted me, she was taking 200 mcg of thyroxine daily yet still suffered a range of symptoms, and her weight, blood pressure and blood cholesterol levels were all too high. (Blood pressure and cholesterol increases are both characteristic of hypothyroidism – see page 185.)

I requested a blood test to assess thyroid function and cholesterol levels. Meg's total cholesterol was 7.2 mmol/L (the normal range is under 5) and her Free T4 (blood thyroxine level) was 21 pmol/L. Her blood pressure was 178/108 – a good, normal blood pressure reading is between 120/80 and 140/90 for her age. As I have already stated, her weight at consultation was 210 lb (95 kg). Meg had been reassured by her doctor that her thyroid function had normalized, as her Free T4 was at 21 (well within the laboratory's normal range of 9–24). Her morning temperature averaged 96.8 °F/36 °C (see page 198).

Diagnosis

So what was wrong? Meg was still experiencing symptoms of hypothyroidism, yet her blood tests appeared normal. I encounter this diagnostic paradox quite frequently. Patients are biochemically euthyroid (normal thyroid), but clinically hypothyroid (showing symptoms of hypothyroidism).

There are two explanations for this phenomenon:

1 The thyroid hormone that is usually measured in the blood and prescribed is named thyroxine (T4). However, T4 converts to T3 (or triiodothyronine), the more chemically active hormone, at cell level. In some cases of hypothyroidism the essential conversion of T4 to T3 is impaired by free radical damage, liver toxicity or enzyme failure. If this poor conversion is present, additional thyroxine may not always be the answer. In the UK the prescription for hypothroidism is thyroxine alone. This is based on the assumption that the thyroxine converts to T3. In the US and many other countries, the prescription protocol is

to combine T3 and T4 or, with mild hypothyroidism, to prescribe animal glandular supplements, as they provide the precursors for *all* the thyroid hormones.

2   The interpretation of the laboratory results should have included Meg's symptom-picture. I do not believe that a blood T4 level can be seen as normal unless the blood improvement is matched by symptom improvement. In Meg's case her blood showed a 'normal' level of 21 for the thyroxine. The question was, just what should her ideal level have been?

Controversy surrounds the question of normal ranges for thyroid hormone testing. Many laboratory workers and doctors insist that two normal ranges should be recognized:

a   A normal range for symptom-free individuals who are not taking thyroxine
b   A normal range for patients who *are* taking thyroxine.

The Free T4 test involves measuring the amount of this hormone in the blood. It follows that a percentage of the thyroxine measured in the blood will include the thyroxine taken each day. With this in mind, it would make sense to have a higher 'normal range' for patients taking thyroxine.

Sir Richard Bayliss (an eminent endocrinologist and author) made a very appropriate comment on this topic during a talk given at the Medical Society of London in January 1995. He stated, 'Certainly it is my experience that patients feel at their best when the free thyroxine level is towards the upper end of the reference range, or marginally above it.'

Thus, in Meg's case, all the evidence suggested that her thyroid was still not doing its job.

Treatment

There is no conflict or risk when patients combine hormone therapy with glandular or nutritional supplements. Indeed, approximately one-third of my hypothyroid patients are taking thyroxine.

Meg was prescribed glandular and nutritional support for her thyroid and adrenals, and after four months her blood thyroxine had increased to 26 pmol/L.

Eight months into the combination treatment, her blood thyroxine was 33 pmol/L and Meg was feeling in her own words '75% better'. At this stage I considered it appropriate for her to commence a more disciplined dieting and exercise programme.

Meg's existing diet was a low-fat, low-sugar diet of around 1,500 calories. She had not exercised for many years. I encouraged her to join a local gym and to swim 3–4 times each week. In addition to a low-carbohydrate diet, I also advised Meg to have a fresh-fruit-and-water-only day every fifth day. I find this plan very useful to 'kick-start' a sluggish metabolism when the overweight is long term. The plan is simple: Fresh fruit only (though no bananas, dried fruit or dates) taken at mealtimes with only bottled mineral water to drink. (Many of my patients find sparkling water more filling.) This regime usually totals 350–500 calories daily, depending on the choice of fruit. Fruit is very filling, offers a useful high-fibre bowel detox, and most patients enjoy the programme. They usually prefer to do their fruit days on their busiest days, as no cooking is required.

Conclusion

Meg is still seeing me, and at her last visit she weighed 160 lb (73 kg), with a BMI of 25. Her ambition is to achieve a weight of around 140 lb (63 kg) with a BMI of 21–22. It is probable that she will not reach this ideal weight for another 6–8 months, making for a total of two years before she will have achieved normal health since the time of our first consultation. This recovery time tends to demonstrate the well-known slow response by the thyroid to any treatment. It is not a gland noted for rapid changes. Patience and persistence are required following satisfactory diagnosis and treatment.

High Blood Pressure and the Thyroid

As Meg's case has shown us, underactive thyroid can have an influence on blood pressure. This can reveal itself in various ways:

1 A reduction in the blood supply to the kidneys can raise blood pressure. This can occur in hypothyroidism as a result of atherosclerosis (narrowing) of the kidney blood vessels.
2 Surgery to treat thyroid enlargement (goitre) can lead to blood pressure increases in proportion to the amount of thyroid gland removed.
3 Operations to remove the thyroid (thyroidectomy) can cause high blood pressure or worsen an existing tendency.
4 There is evidence available to show that patients who are successfully treated for hypothyroidism do not have high blood pressure, as the thyroid therapy reduces the pressure without the need for anti-hypertensive drugs.
5 The increased body weight, fluid retention and raised blood cholesterol that occurs with hypothyroidism can all contribute to high blood pressure.

Cholesterol and the Thyroid

Cholesterol Testing
The link between blood cholesterol levels and thyroid function was first discussed in 1918. It was observed that the blood cholesterol levels in animals decreased when they were given desiccated thyroid.

It was demonstrated in the 1930s that patients with hyperthyroidism frequently showed low blood cholesterol levels (often well below what was considered normal). After surgery to remove part of the thyroid the cholesterol level increased to above normal, suggesting that too much thyroid tissue had been removed, rendering the patient hypothyroid. If the patient was then given thyroid treatment, the cholesterol levels normalized.

All this caused considerable excitement in the 1930s, and many researchers and doctors became convinced that if thyroid hormones controlled the blood cholesterol levels in their patients, measuring the cholesterol offered a very useful test for assessing thyroid function. Dr Broda Barnes, however, found that, 'Blood cholesterol cannot be depended upon as a universal indicator of hypothyroidism.' His research confirmed that, in young patients, the cholesterol level can be normal regardless of thyroid activity, and high cholesterol could not always be demonstrated (see References, *Hypothyroidism – The Unsuspected Illness*).

How Can I Tell If It's a Thyroid Problem?

You may well question the need to suspect an underactive thyroid, and you may feel quite healthy, albeit overweight. If you are simply too heavy without any other symptoms, your thyroid is unlikely to be a cause of your excess weight. But just to be on the safe side, answer the following questions (please note: If your weight gain is recent – in the past 12–18 months – change references to 5 years in this questionnaire to 1 year):

1 Do you have the same energy that you had 5 years ago?
2 Is your concentration as sharp as it was 5 years ago?
3 Is your short-term memory as good as it was 5 years ago?
4 Do you feel at your best on rising?
5 Is your digestion working well and symptom-free?
6 Do you have a backache or neck-ache on rising?
7 Are you generally a 'cold' person, with cold hands and feet?
8 Do you easily become depressed or anxious?

9 Is your libido reduced compared with 5 years ago?
10 Just how much weight have you put on over the previous
  5 years? Is it in excess of 10%?

Results

If you answer 'Yes' for questions 1–5 and 'No' for 6–10, then your thyroid is unlikely to be a factor in your excess weight. If however you have two or more 'No' answers for questions 1–5, and two or more 'Yes' answers for questions 6–10, there is a real chance that your thyroid is contributing to your weight problem.

Self-assessment

In my book *Why Am I So Tired?*, which discusses mild hypothyroidism, there is a chapter entitled 'Diagnosing Your Mild Hypothyroidism'. The strategy for assessing your thyroid activity and diagnosing a depressed or inefficient thyroid consists of:

1 A careful assessment of your symptoms and past history, by use of a questionnaire.
2 Taking your body temperature after waking.

Symptom Questionnaire

I have devised the following questionnaire to help you assess your symptoms and medical history. **Use this questionnaire only as a guide. It is essential you consult a qualified doctor or naturopath before beginning any treatment or supplement programme.**

Complete each of the sections below and then add the results of each section to obtain a total score.

Section A: Past History
Scoring: 10 points for each 'Yes' answer.

1   Is there a history of thyroid disease in your family?
2   Have you at any time required throat or neck surgery
    (e.g. for tonsillitis)?
3   Have you ever been the victim of a road traffic accident
    involving a neck injury (e.g. whiplash)?
4   Have you in the past suffered from any of the following
    conditions: glandular fever, systemic candidiasis, hepatitis,
    chronic fatigue syndrome or anorexia nervosa?
5   Have you a history of chronic constipation?
6   Have you a history of high blood pressure?
7   Have you a history of depression?
8   Have you ever been seriously overweight (e.g. 20% over
    optimal weight)?
9   Have you had a general anaesthetic in the previous
    two years?
10 If you have been pregnant, did any of the following health
    problems occur: Miscarriage, obesity, postnatal depression
    or thyroid imbalance?

TOTAL for Section A: ___ points.

Section B: Current Symptoms
Scoring:
5 points   If the symptom is trivial and/or occasional
10 points   If the symptom is moderate and/or frequent
15 points   If the symptom is severe and/or constant

1   Physical fatigue
2   Poor concentration
3   Poor short-term memory

 4 Depression
 5 Cold extremities (e.g. hands and feet)
 6 Muscle pain and cramping
 7 Generally feeling worse just after waking up
 8 Low libido (sex drive)
 9 Moodiness/irritability
10 Anxiety
11 Symptoms worse with missed meals
12 PMS
13 Heavy periods
14 Constipation
15 Dry skin and/or hair loss
16 Unexplained weight gain
17 Frequent infections (e.g. throat or lung infection)
18 Headaches
19 Catarrhal/nasal congestion
20 Dizziness, poor balance

TOTAL for Section B: ___ points.

Section C: Tests and Treatment
Scoring: 100 points for each 'Yes' answer.

1 Have you had a thyroid hormone blood test over the previous two years, with a Free T4 under 15 pmol/L or a TSH over 4.0 mU/L?
2 Have you in the past needed thyroid surgery or radioactive iodine treatment for 'hyperthyroidism' (overactive thyroid)?
3 Have blood tests shown you to have a raised cholesterol?
4 Is your morning temperature constantly below 97.5 °F (36.4 °C)?

TOTAL for Section C: ___ points.

Analysis

When you have arrived at a grand total by adding your scores for Sections A, B and C together, you can assess the likelihood that you have mild hypothyroidism:

600–800	Almost certain
400–600	Probable
200–400	Possible
0–200	Unlikely

Summary

As I have mentioned above, this type of assessment should only be seen as a rough guide. However, those readers whose scores total over 500 points would be advised to seek professional help from a sympathetic medical doctor or naturopath who is familiar with thyroid disease and treatment. They can then carry out more detailed investigations.

Taking Your Early Morning Temperature

Your normal body temperature on waking, or basal temperature measurement (BTM), has for over 100 years been recognized as a valuable indicator of thyroid activity. (This is why I frequently ask patients if they are a 'cold' or 'warm' person.)

Doctors and other practitioners have observed that patients with a sluggish thyroid have below-normal temperatures. This is not too surprising, as we know that the thyroid has a direct effect on our metabolic rate, and the metabolism has a direct influence on body temperature. Our metabolic rate increases when our temperature increases, and decreases when our temperature falls. A fever, for example, is the body's attempt to increase immune response by raising our temperature.

In the 1940s American doctor Broda Barnes pioneered a systematic method of thyroid diagnosis based on this early-morning temperature evidence. I recommend you try this test, as it is a safe and easy way to assess the efficiency of your thyroid gland.

1 Place a thermometer under your arm as soon as you wake up, and leave it there for 10 minutes (do not get out of bed, or even talk, during this time!).

2 Try to do this at the same time each day.

3 Test for at least three consecutive days.

4 Men can check their temperature on any three days. For women who are menstruating, the temperature is best measured on days 2, 3 and 4 of their period. Before puberty and after the menopause, any three days will suffice.

Some doctors request women to test for 28 days to obtain more accurate average temperatures. This can become rather tedious, and I do find that an average of three days' readings provides sufficient diagnostic information.

Temperatures

The 'normal' under-the-tongue temperature for a healthy person is 98.6 °F or 37 °C. The 'normal' BTM, however, is in the range 97.8–98.2 °F or 36.6–36.8 °C. I have found that temperatures as low as 95.6 °F or 35.4 °C are not unusual in hypothyroid patients.

Dr Barnes held the rather simplistic view that a morning temperature below 97.8 °F/36.6 °C indicated hypothyroidism, while a temperature above 98.2 °F/36.8 °C indicated hyperthyroidism.

However, the BTM is not a definitive test, nor 100 per cent accurate, when used in conjunction with the other methods of diagnosis it is a useful indicator of hypothyroidism and offers a valuable means to monitor progress under treatment. The temperature increase associated with improvement is often evident before there is any symptom relief, and before the levels of the thyroid blood tests show any improvement. Thus it offers a subtle indication of thyroid change.

Lorna's Story

Lorna consulted me with chronic fatigue, poor concentration and short-term memory, overweight, eczema and PMS. Being a student aged 22, these symptoms were causing her and her family great concern, as she had also recently slipped into a depression. Many of Lorna's symptoms had been with her for 7–8 years, and her doctor had decided that the depression was the cause. (It surprises me just how many different symptoms are currently being attributed to depression. In many patients I find that depression is in fact secondary to and caused by other symptoms.) Lorna had declined the offer of anti-depressants, and when she came to see me she was not receiving any treatment.

She enjoyed a sensible, healthy diet of around 2,000 calories per day, and was an occasional, social drinker but not a smoker. Surprisingly for a student, she neither drank tea or coffee nor ate sweets or chocolates.

Examination

Lorna's height was 5 ft 3 in (160 cm) and her weight was 171 lb (77 kg), giving her a BMI of 30.2, or seriously overweight. Her blood pressure was normal, and her early morning basal temperature averaged 96.8 °F (36 °C). She completed the questionnaire (as found on pages 194–97) and came up with a total score of 550 points (in the 'probable' range for mild hypothyroidism).

All the evidence at this point suggested that Lorna had a depressed thyroid function, so blood tests were requested. Although her Free T4 (thyroxine) was within the normal ranges, it was borderline at 10.0 pmol/L. The laboratory that I use recommends a normal range of 9.4–24.0 pmol/L.

Treatment

I prescribed nutritional supplements for Lorna, coupled with thyroid glandular support (bovine). I also recommended regular swimming and walking.

A further blood test was done three months after the first consultation, and the Free T4 was up to 13.0. Lorna was at this point feeling, in her own words 'at least 50% better'. Her weight was 161 lb (73 kg). A further blood test was requested six months after the initial test, and the results showed a Free T4 of 15 pmol/L. Lorna's morning temperatures were averaging 97.4 °F (36.3 °C).

Her energy was now virtually 100%, and she was able to swim non-stop for 60 lengths of the swimming pool. Her weight had dropped to 150 lb (68 kg), with a resulting BMI of 26.8. Lorna only needed to lose another few pounds to be a normal weight for her height.

Significantly, I had not advised Lorna to reduce her food intake. I felt that normalizing her metabolism with thyroid support, and gradually increasing her swimming, would be sufficient to enable her to reduce weight. When students are studying hard it is very important for them to eat a simple but healthy and balanced diet. Calorie-counting and crash-diet programmes are not appropriate when the brain is working at full capacity.

An Ideal Level?

You may ask 'How do I know what is the ideal level for my thyroid hormones?' The British Thyroid Foundation is currently lobbying the Minister of Health to consider a programme of routine thyroid testing for all children when they reach the age of 18 years. This would provide a useful baseline for everyone to compare with any subsequent thyroid changes in later life (assuming that most of us are slim and fit at 18 years old!).

Unfortunately, very few people undergo blood thyroid tests when they are feeling well, so test results usually reflect their symptoms and not the normal thyroid output.

I often request blood tests when patients feel recovered and are quite happy with their symptoms and weight. This may follow 6–9 months of treatment. Such tests usually reflect a normally functioning thyroid, and the results can be used as a guideline for future testing. Although the normal range may be 9 or 10–25, many patients discover that their normal or optimum level of blood thyroxine is, for example, 16 – and if they fall below 16, symptoms can develop.

The average blood thyroxine level for symptom-free individuals is 16.9.

Treating an Underactive Thyroid

Many of my patients, when given a diagnosis of mild hypothyroidism, wrongly assume that after taking thyroid supplements for a few months their weight will automatically normalize. This is not always the case. It is important to balance the metabolism and to raise energy levels, body temperature and blood hormones. However, it is also important to address the two other elements required for lasting weight loss: an appropriate diet to match the patient's lifestyle and activity level, and a well-thought out and agreeable exercise programme. I tell my patients with low-grade thyroid activity that weight loss is next to impossible, even with a suitable diet and regular exercise (if they have the energy), when their thyroid is so depressed. They are lucky just to maintain their current weight.

Just as there are three elements required before a diagnosis can be made (i.e. blood results, temperature and symptoms), I believe that there are also three treatment elements before a hypothyroid patient can lose weight and maintain an ideal weight:

1 Symptom relief and metabolic efficiency
2 Appropriate diet
3 Exercise.

Thyroid Supplements for Symptom Relief

Raw Glandular Therapy

Animal tissue concentrates, also termed 'protomorphogens' or 'organ-specifics', have been in use for thousands of years. The like-cures-like basis of this therapy rests on the assumption that by using animal glands, the appropriate nutrient proportions can be provided as are found in our own organs and glands. The glandular preparations in current use are called 'raw' because no heat is used in their processing. The glands are taken from Canadian corn-fed cattle. After removal, the glands are de-fatted and kept frozen until processed.

The critics of raw glandulars (who use the derogatory term 'cow parts') argue that they fail to be clinically effective for two reasons:

1 The material contained in the glands is reduced to basic amino acids (the building blocks of protein) in the process of digestion, and therefore does not possess any specific therapeutic value. The glandular detractors argue that patients who take glandular supplements would obtain the same 'benefits' by eating any type of protein (e.g. fish, meat, cheese or eggs).
2 The other argument against tissue specifics in therapy claims that unless proteins are broken down into simple amino acids they cannot be absorbed from the gut and passed into the bloodstream, as they would be too large.

There is evidence available to show that when enzymes and proteins are eaten and absorbed through the gut lining, approximately 50% passes into the blood. Significantly, this is in the form of molecules that have been reduced to amino acids. Leon Chaitow states in his book *The Raw Materials of Health*: 'Furthermore, and of critical significance to the concept of using specific organs and glands in therapy, it is known that at least 20% of these unchanged (by digestion) protein molecules retain their original characteristics.'

It seems likely, therefore, that when raw glandular supplements are properly prepared from healthy, free-range animals, they provide a specific therapeutic value for the gland that is targeted. The nutritional make up of the glands and organs of animals are chemically very similar to their human counterparts. It follows, therefore, that the specific nutritional constituents which are provided by such a system will be in the optimum ratios and quantities.

When patients are prescribed thyroxine for their underactive thyroid, subsequent blood tests usually show that their blood thyroxine (Free T4) level has increased. This is not too surprising, but the improvement in the blood is not always paralleled by symptom improvement. Furthermore, taking thyroxine does not guarantee an increase in the efficiency of a patient's thyroid gland. In fact, by artificially introducing a hormone the gland concerned can become *less* efficient, thus reducing its output. For this reason the prescription for thyroxine in the UK is a free prescription, as a dependency is quickly created and the prescribed thyroxine is required for the rest of the patient's life.

With the use of thyroid tissue supplements, however, the blood thyroxine improves as a direct result of the patient's thyroid becoming more efficient. When this improvement leads to symptom relief, and blood test results improve, the thyroid tissue supplements can be discontinued, or continued on only a low-maintenance dose. The latter usually applies to very elderly patients or patients who have experienced symptoms for many years.

An Appropriate Diet

When I am treating patients with mild hypothyroidism I do not always prescribe a special diet from day one. There are several reasons for this.

Overweight thyroid patients are usually fatigued and depressed. They are often frustrated and very disappointed with their failure to obtain results with special diets. This can be particularly upsetting when many other dieters seem to lose weight following similar diets. For this reason I do not consider that it is always wise to present such patients with yet another special diet. I prefer to wait until their symptoms begin to improve before we talk about food and food selection.

Another reason for my misgivings over handing out a diet sheet at our first meeting is simply that diets do not initially work with hypothyroid patients. I usually tell them that they are very lucky if they can 'hold' their weight with their underfunctioning thyroid.

When patients begin to feel a little more vital (usually after 3–4 months of treatment), I prescribe a low-carbohydrate diet as outlined in Chapter 2.

Exercise

In my experience, fatigued, depressed, overweight hypothyroid patients do not follow exercise programmes, simply because they do not have the energy, motivation or patience to follow any programme that requires vitality, time and discipline.

However, again after 3–4 months of treatment I usually prescribe the final element of exercise (see Chapter 11 for details).

Tom's Story

Consultation

When Tom first consulted me he stated that the only time in his life when he'd been a normal weight was as a baby. Since the age of 7 he had been overweight. At the time he came to see me he weighed 322 lb (146 kg); at 5 ft 10 in (178 cm) this gave him a BMI of 46 – putting Tom into the 'dangerously overweight' category.

Excess weight was not Tom's only concern. He also suffered from fatigue and poor memory and concentration, which caused him to be moody, irritable and depressed. He defined his condition as being 'woolly-headed'. Other symptoms included dry skin, low libido (sex drive) and a very poor resistance to infections, which he described as 'one cold after another', usually leading to chest infections. Tom made a point of telling me how irritable and tired he always felt on waking. His colleagues at work were so accustomed to his morning moods that they usually delayed any decision-making or discussions with him until after lunch.

With no family history of obesity and with Tom's general good health (he had never had surgery or been hospitalized in his adult life), the cause or causes of his obesity were not immediately obvious. However, two clues became apparent as I questioned him. His tonsils had been removed at the age of 6, only a few months prior to the onset of his rapid weight gain. In addition, his older brother had recently been diagnosed as hypothyroid.

I believe that a causative link exists between throat surgery, injury or infections in early life and adult hypothyroidism. Many patients comment that their symptoms developed shortly after a brush with tonsillitis, whiplash injury (as after a road traffic accident), heavy dental work or throat surgery. It is entirely possible that these conditions can compromise the circulation to the thyroid gland.

Blood Tests

I requested a full thyroid profile blood test. Tom's results gave a figure of 13 pmol/L for the blood thyroxine (Free T4), the normal range (for the lab used) being 11.5–22.5. As discussed, even though a patient's results may be within the normal recommended range, it cannot be assumed that all is indeed normal. Tom was 42 and his ideal level for blood thyroid should have been 16–20.

Temperature

As mentioned earlier, many patients with mild hypothyroidism have a low body temperature. For many years the 'basal temperature measurement' or BTM has been seen as a valuable indicator of thyroid activity. Our metabolic rate directly influences our temperature, and a depressed thyroid will slow the metabolism. The ideal temperature on waking is 97.8–98.2 °F (36.5–36.8 °C). Tom's morning temperatures averaged 96.5 °F (35.9 °C).

Diagnosis

Tom thus met the three criteria for a diagnosis of mild hypothyroidism: his symptoms, morning temperature, and blood test results.

Diet

When patients book for a consultation to see me, my secretary always requests a brief written health history, details of any prescription drugs and supplements being taken, and a three-day record of all food and drink consumed. Having this information available at the consultation allows more time to discuss symptoms and treatment. Many patients with mild hypothyroidism suffer with a very poor short-term memory. The request to write their health history serves as a useful memory-jogger, and names and dosages of prescription drugs can easily be forgotten if not written down.

Tom's diet was difficult to fault. This I find, is so often the case when obesity is a symptom of an underlying health problem rather than a result of overeating or taking too little exercise. Tom was following a low-fat diet with a calorie count of approximately 2,000 calories a day. Unfortunately, though, his diet included such foods as potatoes, bread, cereals, crisps, ice-cream, lemonade, meat pies and other carbohydrates.

Treatment

I prescribed two supplements for Tom: T Lyph™, a product supplied by Nutri Ltd (see Resources page 253), and is made from animal thyroids, and Thyro-Complex™. Also produced by Nutri Ltd, this supplement, which I formulated, provides all the nutrients required for optimum thyroid metabolism. The constituents are:

L-Tyrosine	L-Carnitine	DL-Phenylalanine
Dong Quai	Iodine (Kelp)	Liquorice Root
Vitamin A (palmite)	Folic Acid	Vitamin B_1 (thiamine HCl)
Vitamin B_2 (riboflavin)	Vitamin B_3 (niacin)	Vitamin B_6 (pyridoxine HCL)
Vitamin C	Vitamin E	Selenium (aspartate)
Zinc (picolinate)	Calcium (aspartate)	Magnesium (aspartate)
Copper (chelate)	Manganese (chelate)	

Conclusion

Tom has lost 42 lb (19 kg) in 10 months. The combination of thyroid support, dieting and exercise (mainly swimming) is beginning to work for him. Perhaps more important for Tom than his weight is his general improvement in energy and mood. He is beginning to actually enjoy driving to work each morning, and his colleagues now talk to him before the lunch break. It may well require another 12–18 months of treatment before he achieves an ideal weight, but the chief cause of his symptoms has been identified and the treatment components are now in place and working for him.

Chapter Summary

1 A mildly underactive thyroid is a commonly missed cause of stubborn overweight.

2 Other symptoms will usually be present, including mental and physical fatigue, poor quality hair and skin, low blood sugar, depression, muscle pain and stiffness, and reduced libido.

3 The standard medical blood tests for thyroid function are designed only to identify and diagnose severe thyroid problems. Mild thyroid deficiencies can therefore be missed. Diagnosis should be based on three clues: symptoms, body temperature, and laboratory tests.

4 Even when the thyroid is stable and symptom-relief is beginning, weight loss is not automatic. However, as your thyroid improves, diets and exercise programmes will become more successful.

5 Many individuals who are already taking thyroxine remain fatigued and overweight. Even when you are told that your blood tests are 'normal', do not give up, look again! Nutritional or glandular supplements can provide beneficial 'fine-tuning' to speed-up symptom-relief and weight loss.

6 The improvement in vitality with correct treatment will encourage more activity and exercise, breaking the vicious circle of weight, fatigue and more weight.

7 When you are fit and slim and your symptoms have improved, request another thyroid function test. This will provide you with accurate evidence of your 'normal' hormone levels, which can be relied upon for future comparisons and reference.

Part Three

Helping Yourself and
Those You Care About

CHAPTER TEN

Children and Overweight

I shall begin this chapter with a few statistics. I know that many of us view statistics with derision, doubt or disbelief. Yet the evidence of our own eyes confirms that we are seeing more and more overweight children in the shops, the schools and on the streets.

So here are the statistics. These are American figures, but UK children are catching up fast! (These statistics relate to obesity – that is, children with a BMI of 30 or over. The number of children who are 'simply' overweight is far higher.)

1 Over the last 40 years, there has been a 50% increase in childhood obesity in the US.
2 Approximately 20% of all American children (12 million) are overweight.
3 Only 1% of obese children have a medical condition that causes their overweight. So where does the weight come from?

Inheritance or Environment?

Controversy exists over the possible causes of childhood overweight. It is generally accepted that genetics (inherited factors) and environment (activity, diet, etc.) share responsibility for the current problem of overweight children.

Valuable studies in Denmark (where the records of children's natural and adoptive parents are particularly comprehensive) point to childhood obesity in adopted children correlating to their natural parents and not their adoptive ones, suggesting that inheritance is more likely to cause overweight than the pattern of a child's upbringing and diet.

However, the environment lobby also has a strong case. American children watch TV an average of three hours each day. This does not include the time spent playing computer games. In the pre-TV age of the 1940s and 1950s, children were encouraged to 'go out and play' if dinner wasn't ready or if they were bored. Now the advice is often 'go watch TV'.

Many paediatricians and naturopaths consider that childhood overweight and obesity result from an imbalance between the energy input (food) and energy output (exercise): Too much of the former and too little of the latter. In conclusion, genes are generally blamed for up to 25–40% of obesity, with 60–75% a result of environmental factors.

Eating Habits

Our pattern of eating has changed over the last 20–30 years. Instead of the traditional three meals per day. Many households have six or seven snack meals each day. A high percentage of families rarely eat around a table together. Eating in front of the TV or even the computer has become an increasingly common phenomenon. Unfortunately snacks, are frequently convenience foods which tend to be high in carbohydrates, saturated fats and sugar. Pizzas, sandwiches, rolls, burgers, biscuits and cakes are easier to eat than homemade soups, casseroles and roasts, and certainly much easier to prepare and serve.

According to a study of 800 British children questioned in 2001 by the Doctor-Patient Partnership (a branch of the British Medical Association), 200 of the children questioned admitted to not having breakfast at home, but eating crisps and sweets for breakfast on their way to school.

In the US, the link between sugar consumption in soft drinks and obesity among children has been studied. Hundreds of children were closely studied for two years for the amount of soft drinks that they consumed. (The drinks included cola, lemonade, sugared fruit drinks and juices, and various sodas.) The report, also published in the UK medical journal *The Lancet*, concluded that 'The odds of becoming obese increased significantly with each additional daily serving of sugar-sweetened drink.'

More than 57% of the children in this study increased their consumption over the two-year period, 25% by as much as two or more additional cans per day. The consumption of soft drinks has almost doubled among children in the US over the past decade. When this is converted to sugar-intake, the consumption of sugar by the average American teenager now amounts to 15–20 additional teaspoons a day from soft drinks alone, compared with 10 years ago.

Childhood Overweight – The Consequences

Readers may wonder why a chapter on overweight children is included in a book dealing with the health causes of excess weight in adults. But being obese or simply overweight as a child carries a long-term health risk into adult life.

Studies have confirmed that excessive weight in children and adolescents increases the risk of various health problems in adulthood, irrespective of whether the obese children grow into obese or slender adults. A normal-weight adult who was overweight or obese as a child is more likely to suffer poor health than an adult whose weight has been normal since birth.

One important study was written up in the *American Heart Journal* in 1971 by Dr G. E. Burch. He demonstrated that when animals are overfed when young, their fat cells increase faster than normal. When growth and cell increase has ceased (as animals – or people – reach adulthood), the number of fat cells remains constant throughout the remainder of life. This means that a child who has laid down too many fat cells can reach adulthood with more than three times as many as someone who has not been overweight as a child. If these fat cells are subsequently used (that is, filled), adult obesity results.

So what are the long-term health risks for overweight or obese children? Unfortunately this is a long list, including the following physical and psychological conditions.

Physical
- High blood pressure
- Diabetes
- High blood cholesterol
- High blood triglycerides
- Menstrual imbalances
- Early hypothyroidism
- Joint disorders
- Sleep apnoea
- Asthma
- Cardio-vascular disorders

Psychological
- Low self-esteem
- Low confidence
- Social isolation

- Poor academic performance
- Dislike of sport
- Eating disorders

Defining 'Overweight' in Children

As for adults, the Body Mass Index (BMI) is generally seen as the most reliable indicator of childhood overweight and obesity. (See page 7 for how one's BMI is calculated.)

Research defines overweight and obesity using the following BMI levels for children of different ages:

Age	Overweight (boys)	Overweight (girls)	Obese (boys)	Obese (girls)
2–5 years	15	14.8	20	19.8
5–10 years	14.3	14.2	19.3	19.2
10–15 years	19	19.2	24	24.2
15–18 years	23.3	24.2	28.3	29.2
18 years+	25	25	30	30

Treating Overweight Children

There is one essential difference between overweight adults and overweight children: Children are still growing.

An overweight 15-year-old boy who can avoid further weight gain for 12 months may no longer be overweight at 16 years. He may be 2 inches taller and have quite a normal BMI.

An acceptable aim for overweight children is to attempt to slow or stop their weight gain, and allow them to 'grow into' their existing weight. It is not always appropriate or wise to subject a child to the discipline of a low-calorie or reduced-food weight-loss programme. Such a regime can easily be interpreted by the child as a form of punishment, a view that will only encourage him or her to rebel against the diet. This particularly as the other major component of weight loss – energy expenditure or exercise – may not be fully utilized.

Exercise

It has been stated by many doctors and naturopaths that lack of exercise is the chief cause of childhood overweight. The 'couch potato' syndrome has been well defined and discussed. We all agree that modern children rarely walk to school anymore, their school sports have been reduced and they spend too much time watching TV. They have become computer screen spectators when they should be participants. So what can be done to persuade a child to do more exercise? The following ideas may help.

Begin by sharing activities with your children. Sweat with them, whether walking, jogging, running, swimming or cycling.

Consider introducing new sporting activities, with the inducement of lessons in dance, skating, horse-riding, golf, badminton, etc.

Involve your children in sporting activities and reduce their role as spectators. This will assist with weight control, provide you with time to talk with them and – perhaps most important – minimize their time spent slumped in front of the TV or computer screen.

Encourage your child to use a stationary bike while watching TV.

Do not criticize a child's efforts to exercise, or set too strict a regime.

Avoid blaming your child for being overweight. They will already feel bad about their appearance.

Children see their parents as role models, so set a good example. You'll have a stronger case for encouraging or motivating your children to lose weight when you yourself are healthy and active. Motivation by example must play a major part in helping your child.

Diets?

I do not always recommend diets for overweight children. They are rarely followed and, as I have said, actual weight loss is not the chief aim here. Encourage family meals around the table, forbid snacks in bedrooms and in front of the TV. Avoid between-meal snacks and sugar- and fat-rich foods. Introduce variety into your catering and attempt to use wholegrain cereals and good-quality proteins. Always have fresh fruit available, and introduce the Mediterranean idea of a salad course.

Healthy eating and activity patterns need to be established, then perhaps overweight children will not always end up as overweight adults.

CHAPTER ELEVEN

Exercise and Your Weight

The link between exercise and weight loss is controversial.

I often remind my patients of the 'trilogy' of causes that needs to be successfully addressed before lasting weight-loss can be achieved: diet, exercise, and metabolism. Every chapter so far has looked at the various metabolic causes of overweight, and the question of diets has also been discussed. Now let's take a look at exercise.

Patients' Objections

Many of my patients are initially antagonistic to the idea of regular exercise. It may be worthwhile to list the reasons that are offered by those who do not exercise, or do not want to exercise:

1 'I am too old for that sort of thing.'
2 'I hate gyms, they are boring, embarrassing and expensive.'
3 'I haven't time to exercise.'
4 'Exercise just makes you sweat and lose fluid, which you quickly replace.'

5 'Exercise can damage muscles and joints and can give people heart attacks.'

6 'I am far too embarrassed to strip off in public in my present shape and weight.'

7 'Exercise just increases your appetite and makes you eat more afterwards.'

8 'I have a problem with my ankles/knee/back/etc. and exercise makes it worse.'

9 'I have exercised every weekend for months and it hasn't made much difference to my weight.'

10 'I exercise enough already, with two young children and a house to run.'

11 'I just lack the required discipline to exercise regularly.'

12 'I have been advised not to exercise as I have asthma/diabetes/high blood pressure/low blood sugar/epilepsy, etc.'

As this is essentially a problem-solving book, I shall briefly respond to these 12 typical arguments against taking regular exercise to help them lose weight.

1. Too Old?

You can exercise at any age. Remember the formula for the predicted maximum heart rate (see page 227) and listen to your body. You can safely walk and swim well into your nineties.

2. Gyms

You do not need to attend a gym, though they offer a variety of facilities. And yes, they can be boring, although a jacuzzi, sauna or swim can break the monotony. Local council health-centre gyms can be cheap, and make you feel less like you're on show.

3. Time to Exercise

This can be a problem, as a full visit to a gym or swimming pool needs 60–90 minutes. However, many centres are now open from

7 a.m. to midnight. Some of my patients call into the gym or pool on their way to work, which is a very good way to start the day!

4. Sweating and Exercise
As you will read later in this chapter, there is more to regular exercise than fluid loss.

5. Exercise and Muscle Damage
Self-assessment, self-awareness, sensible 'warm-up' sessions and a personalized selection of exercises will all serve to reduce the risk of damage to your muscles and health.

6. Embarrassment
Although some trendy sports clubs have a fashion-show atmosphere, you can exercise in loose-fitting, casual clothes. Don't be afraid to do a 'consumer check' on your local facilities and find a gym or club that suits you.

7. Appetite and Exercise
Our appetite is mainly influenced by our blood sugar level. You should not exercise on an empty stomach. Blood sugar awareness and exercise is discussed later in this chapter, but for now just note that light to moderate exercise can in fact depress the appetite.

8. Joint Problems and Exercise
You may need to tailor your exercises or sport to your problem. Non-weight-bearing exercises (such as swimming or cycling) may be one way to avoid ankle, knee and low back aggravation. Appropriate exercise should in fact help *ease* your joint problems rather than exacerbate them.

9. Regularity of Exercise
Once-a-week exercise routines, or workouts at weekends only, are just not sufficient to have an impact on your weight. Little and often is preferable to occasional and prolonged when considering exercise.

10. Enough Exercise Already!

Working hard looking after a family or a home may not constitute good exercise. A regular break from such a routine to exercise in a different environment may improve your physical and mental health.

11. Discipline

As with any routine, self-discipline is essential if you are to follow a regular exercise or sport regime successfully. The discipline factor is probably one of the chief attractions of a sports club or gym. Paying a subscription is an excellent inducement for regular use, and professional sports trainers should be available to advise. Exercising with a colleague or friend may also help you keep to your routine, which once established (particularly if it is enjoyable) will be easier to maintain.

12. Existing Health Problems

As far as I am aware, there are no health problems or diseases for which exercise is contra-indicated. However, those people with high blood pressure and serious varicose veins, heart or lung conditions, or if doubt exists as to other risk-factors, you should consult your doctor. Gentle exercise is usually recommended for convalescence and many health problems. Some of our top sportsmen and -women have diabetes or disabilities.

Before Exercising

Always ensure that you have an empty bladder before you exercise. Do not eat a heavy meal or drink alcohol just before exercising. Make sure that you have mineral water available to sip during your routine at the gym. Start slowly and carefully. Remember the golden rule: If it hurts – stop! Stop also if you feel dizzy, faint or unusually breathless. If any of these symptoms continues or re-occurs, seek medical advice.

Using Gym Equipment

When you join a gym you should not be allowed to use any of the equipment until you have had an induction session with a trainer. During this session the trainer will work out your heart and pulse rate. He or she will listen to your worries and fears, and will work out an exercise programme designed specifically for you. You will be shown how to use the equipment safely, and your progress will be reviewed and programme adjusted after about six weeks. In well-run gyms, a trainer should be available at all times to help members with any problems and to watch that members use the equipment correctly and do not slip into any bad habits that will cause problems in the future.

The Dangers of Running

Dr Henry Solomon, author of *The Exercise Myth*, makes the following observations:

> Running injuries are especially common because of the punishing force your body has to take. The impact on each jogging step is two to three times your body weight. On average, your feet will strike the ground 800–1,000 times per mile. If you are a 150-pound runner, you generate and must endure at least 120 tons of force per mile – a marathon runner may easily face more than 3,000 tons in a single race.

On a less technical note, runners in a road race held each year in Atlanta, Georgia, when questioned, reported the following traumas over the previous year of running:

- 35% had suffered running injuries
- 61% had suffered dog bites
- 12% had collided with bicycles or cars.

More than 100 were injured by thrown objects, including cans, bottles, ice, liquid and – in one case – a bag of rocks!

Non-competitive running or jogging, wearing appropriate footwear, preferably done on grass rather than on roads, can, however, have a useful role to play in weight-loss programmes.

Why Exercise?

Books written on health and weight usually include a chapter on exercise. However, there exists a great deal of public confusion over several key questions on exercise. These questions involve which exercise to choose, and the duration, intensity and frequency of exercise necessary. You may ask at this point 'Why exercise at all – why not just diet and lose weight without so much effort?' A tempting thought. Let me respond by quoting *Medical Applications of Clinical Nutrition*:

> The relative contribution of physical inactivity and excessive calorie intake to obesity are clear. In the past, it was generally accepted that the obese condition was the result of excessive food intake. Clearly then, the effective approach to weight control would be some form of caloric restriction through dieting. However this view of obesity is overtly simplistic, as available evidence indicates that excess weight-gain throughout life often closely parallels reduced physical activity rather than an increased calorific intake.

The evidence supporting the view that a desirable body weight can be achieved and maintained with the use of regular exercise is clear and well established.

So the real question isn't whether or not to exercise, but 'What, when, and how to exercise?'

What Exercise?

Exercises fall naturally into three main groups:

1 Recreational games and sports
   This is a huge group including such activities as golf, tennis, surfing, horse-riding, etc. These activities are not easy to evaluate in terms of calories, but they can certainly be part of your programme to reduce fat and maintain fitness.
2 General exercises
   These are usually aerobic activities ('aerobic' means exercise that demands and increases oxygen use). These type of exercises usually involve the large muscles of the body in the thighs, buttocks, abdomen and back. Examples include cycling, swimming, running, skipping, etc.
3 Specific repetitive exercise
   Sometimes termed 'circuit-work'. These involve short (30-minutes+), frequent sessions of high-intensity strength training exercises, usually in a gym, though circuit training can be done at home.

When Should You Exercise?

How often should you exercise, and for how long each time? Two valid questions. A few facts and figures may be useful here.

Each pound of fat contains approximately 3,500 kcal. This can seem a daunting amount when you consider that in order to lose just one pound of body weight you would need to:

walk briskly for 12 hours
play golf for 15 hours
swim for 6 hours
chop wood for 7 hours
run 35 miles.

If you are planning to lose 30–40 pounds, the prospect of engaging in anywhere near this much exercise may seem painfully impossible. The key to successful weight loss through exercise, however, is that the effects are *cumulative*. For example:

One game of golf each week would equal approximately 700 kcal. This works out to a pound in weight lost every 5 weeks, or 10 pounds a year.

It must also be remembered that the heavier the person exercising, the higher the energy cost or calories used.

To return to duration and frequency, research studies into the ideal or optimal exercise frequency has shown that at least three sessions a week are needed to have a significant impact on body weight. Training twice a week was shown to have little or no effect on body weight. As for duration, the recommended amount is around 30 minutes of moderate to vigorous training (or running, swimming or cycling) at each session, to give a calorie use of around 350 kcal per session.

How Should You Exercise?

Exercise intensity, not surprisingly, equates most directly to weight loss. For over 40 years, exercise intensity has been correlated with heart rate as follows:

Maximum Heart Rate (MHR) = 220 minus your age.

So, for example, the MHR for someone 50 years old would be 220–50, or 170.

Fortunately, exercise that gets your heart rate up to 60–80% of your MHR is considered ideal for fitness improvement and weight loss. For our 50-year-old, this would mean a heart rate of 102–136 beats per minute.

If you use a gym, you will probably be supplied with a heart-rate monitor. This is worn like a belt around the chest, and senses your heart rate, which is either beamed to a special watch you can wear or to the piece of equipment you are currently exercising on. With modern gym equipment you can programme the machine by providing your age, weight, exercise duration and your maximum pulse rate; a programme is then set for your requirements.

Some exercise gurus advocate an upper MHR of twice your resting pulse rate, or even $2^1/4$ times your resting rate. For the 50-year-old with a resting rate of perhaps 80 this would offer what I would consider an excessively high MHR of 160–180 beats per minute.

General Rules

Pre-Exercise Check
Before commencing an exercise programme, see your doctor or natural health practitioner to have your blood pressure, joint health and general health checked.

Clothing
Wear loose-fitting clothing and good trainers. It's important not to get too cold, so wear layers.

Warm-Up (4–5 minutes)
It is essential to warm up before exercise to prepare your body (especially your muscles). This will loosen and mobilize your joints, warm up your muscles and increase your heart rate gradually. Five minutes on a stationary bike is a simple warm-up method; running on the spot or brisk walking will also do the job.

Cool-Down (4–5 minutes)
This should be a repeat of the warm-up. This will reduce blood congestion and cramp in your legs, and lessen the risk of next-day muscle ache.

Stretching (3–4 minutes)

This important component of your exercise session should be done twice – after the warm-up and after your cool-down. It increases muscle and joint flexibility and improves circulation to the muscles. Stretching after the warm-up helps you avoid muscle damage.

Do the stretching in a gentle, slow manner, and hold each stretch for as long as indicated below. Breathe normally and do not jerk your limbs or muscles.

1. HAMSTRING STRETCH

Standing erect, place your right foot forward approximately 12 inches (30 cm) in front of you. Lean forward from the waist and gently lean on your left thigh with both hands until you feel the stretch behind your right thigh. Keep the right knee slightly flexed. Hold for 10–12 seconds, then switch legs.

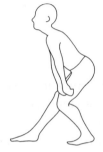

2. CALF STRETCH

Stand erect with your right foot in front of your left approximately 15 inches (38 cm) apart, feet pointing forward. Bend your right (forward) knee slightly, arms outstretched in front of you, keeping the knee over the instep, press the heel of your left leg to the floor and feel the calf stretch. Hold for 10–12 seconds, then switch legs.

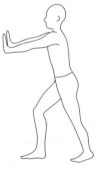

3. QUADRICEP STRETCH

Facing a wall, place your right hand against it, arm straight. With your left hand, grasp your left ankle as you flex your left leg behind you. Keep your right leg slightly bent. Gently pull your left foot towards your buttocks, keeping your knees together.

Hold for 10–12 seconds, then switch legs.

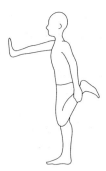

4. SHOULDER STRETCH (1)

Stand erect, clasp your hands together over your head and gently push your hands backwards. Keep looking ahead and maintain a comfortable posture.

Hold for 10–12 seconds.

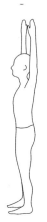

5. SHOULDER STRETCH (2)

Stand erect, clasping your hands behind your back. Remain erect and gently raise your clenched hands without bending forward.

Hold for 10–12 seconds.

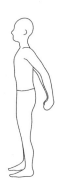

6. BACK STRETCH (1)
Lie on your back and pull your legs to your chest gently, hands holding your thighs.
Hold for 10–12 seconds.

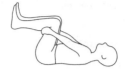

7. BACK STRETCH (2)
This is known as the Cat Stretch. On your hands and knees, arch your back.
Repeat 10–12 times.

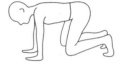

8. WHOLE-BODY STRETCH
Lying on your back, reach your arms above your head and attempt to stretch your whole body. Breathe slowly and deeply; hold for 25–30 seconds. Slowly relax your arms to your sides.

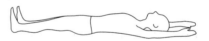

Summary

Assuming you have allowed up to 45 minutes for your exercise session, here's how it should all fit in:

Warm-Up	4–5 minutes
Stretching	3–4 minutes
Full Exercise Session (circuit work in the gym, brisk walking, cycling, jogging, etc.)	20 minutes
Cool-Down	4–5 minutes
Stretching	3–4 minutes
Finish up with a short visit to the sauna, jacuzzi or pool (optional).	

Conclusion

Regular exercise is an important part of anyone's weight-loss programme. Be patient with yourself; it may be 6–8 weeks before you notice any real change. Aside from exercise sessions 3–4 times a week, use stairs instead of lifts and walk or cycle rather than always taking the car or public transport.

Another of the many benefits of exercise as part of a weight-loss plan that includes dieting is that it can provide protection against lean muscle tissue loss, which can occur with dieting alone.

Glossary

Adrenal Glands	Two glands, located adjacent to the top of each kidney. Consisting of two portions, the cortex and the medulla. The cortex secretes cortisol (hydrocortisone), cortisone and adrenal androgens. The androgens serve as precursors to testosterone and oestrogens. The medulla secretes adrenaline (epinephrine) and nor-adrenaline (norepinephrine).
Adrenaline	Also known as epinephrine. A hormone produced by the adrenal glands to facilitate sudden physical activity in an emergency, and to raise the blood sugar level.
Agoraphobia	An anxiety disorder caused by fear of open spaces and crowded public places.
Alzheimer's Disease	Premature senility. Symptoms include confusion, memory failure, speech and movement difficulties, restlessness and loss of intelligence and judgement.

Amenorrhoea	The absence of menstruation.
Amino Acid	The components or building blocks of proteins. More than 100 occur in nature. The *essential* amino acids that must be obtained in our diet are histidine, isoleucine, leucine, lysine, methionine, phenyl-alamine, threonine, tryptophan and valine.
Anaemia	A low level of blood haemoglobin. Causes include a reduction in red cell production, increased red cell destruction, or blood loss. Classification is determined by the haemoglobin level and by the red cell size. There exists many different named anaemias, defined usually by their cause.
Anorexia	Condition caused by a prolonged refusal to eat and characterized by emaciation, cessation of periods, neurosis and fear of obesity. Self-induced vomiting and starvation can require hospitalization. Usually found in young women.
Antioxidant	Nutrients that protect against free radical damage. These antioxidants include vitamin A, C and E, Co-enzyme Q10, milk thistle, selenium, bioflavonoids, quercetin, pynogenal and sulphur containing amino acids and ginkgo biloba.
	Synthetic or natural substances that are added to rubber, paints, vegetable oils and prepared foods to prevent or delay the deterioration by the action of oxygen are also termed antioxidants.
Artheroma	An abnormal build-up of fat in an arterial wall.

Arthritis	Inflammation of joints, usually with pain and swelling.
Atherosclerosis	A disorder of the arteries involving a thickening of the blood vessel walls and a subsequent narrowing of the arteries, resulting in reduced blood flow. Atherosclerosis is a type of arteriosclerosis.
Autism	Mental disorder characterized by poor communication skills, delusions, hallucinations and a withdrawal from reality. Patients are usually totally self-centred.
Auto-immune Disease	Disorder caused as a result of the immune response being directed against the body's own tissues. SLE (Lupus), rheumatoid arthritis, diabetes and hypothyroidism have been classified as auto-immune diseases. The precise cause is not known.
Autonomic Nervous System	A part of the nervous system that regulates non-voluntary functions, including the heart muscle, the intestines and the endocrine glands. It divides into the sympathetic and the parasympathetic branches.
Barnes Temperature Test	A thyroid function test designed by Dr Broda Barnes. This basal temperature test involves a minimum of three on-waking underarm temperature checks. Low temperature levels can be found in mild hypothyroidism, and other disorders.
Basal Temperature Measurement (BTM)	The temperature taken in the morning after sleep and before any activity, including moving, talking, eating, drinking or smoking.

Beta-carotene	A red or orange pro-vitamin that is converted in the body to vitamin A.
Body Mass Index (BMI)	Recommended weight/height ratio. Calculated by dividing your weight in kilograms by the square of your height in metres. A healthy BMI is usually 20–25.
Brown Fat	A type of fat that surrounds the kidneys, heart and adrenal glands. It is also found around the neck and upper spine. Its two chief functions are temperature and weight control. Brown fat accounts for around 10% of the body's fat and it decreases with age.
Bulimia	Insatiable food craving. Binge-eating is often followed by abdominal pain and self-induced vomiting. Unlike anorexia, weight loss does not always occur.
Candidiasis	An infection caused by *Candida albicans*. Symptoms can include nappy (diaper) rash, vaginitis, thrush (vaginal or oral) and pruritus.
Carnitine	An amino-acid, also named vitamin Bt. It is used to reduce blood fat levels and heart disorders being called the 'fat-burner'. Found mainly in red meat, it requires the co-factors iron and vitamin C to prevent a deficiency.
Cholesterol	A fat-soluble substance occurring in animal fats, oils and egg yolks. Found in the bile, blood, brain tissue, liver, kidneys, adrenal glands and nerves. Precursor of steroid and sex hormones including cortisol, cortisone, DHEA, progesterone, oestrogen and testosterone. Cholesterol

can crystallize in the gall bladder to form gall stones. Only 20% of the total cholesterol is dietary, the remaining 80% being produced by the liver.

Coeliac Disease
A disorder caused by an intolerance of gluten (a substance found chiefly in wheat). Also known as non-tropical sprue. Symptoms include bulky, foul-smelling, large stools, weight loss and multiple nutrient-deficiency signs. Avoidance of wheat and other cereals leads to rapid symptom improvement.

Corticosteroids
The hormones associated with the adrenal cortex. Grouped as glucocorticoids (cortisol and corticosterone) and mineralocorticoids (aldosterone). Functions include control or influence of carbohydrate and protein metabolism, fluid balance, circulation system, the skeletal muscles and the kidneys and other organs.

Cortisol (Hydrocortisone)
A steroid hormone produced by the adrenal cortex. Functions include glucose metabolism and protein and fat regulation. It assists in regulation of the immune system.

Cortisone
A steroid hormone involved in carbohydrate and protein regulation. It can be converted into cortisol. However, most of the cortisone found in the body is formed from cortisol.

Desiccated Thyroid
Dried animal thyroid. Perhaps the oldest form of specific thyroid therapy, now largely replaced by raw glandular therapy.

DHEA (Dehydroepiandrosterone)	A 'mother' hormone, made from cholesterol and released by the adrenal glands. The precursor hormone of many steroid and sex hormones.
Dysbiosis	A word used to describe a gradual breakdown of the body's health and balance, 'dys' meaning faulty and 'bios' life or growth.
Dysmenorrhoea	Painful periods, usually causing abdominal and spinal pain.
Ectomorph	*See* Somatotypes.
EFAs (Essential Fatty Acids)	These are fatty acids that cannot be synthesized by human metabolism and must therefore be obtained via food and drink.
Electrocardiogram (ECG)	A record of the electric activity of the heart muscle.
ELISA Test (Enzyme-Linked Immunosorbent Assay)	A blood test that can be used to identify food sensitivities. Food specific antibodies (IgGs) are measured when the blood contacts a panel of foods.
Endocrine System	A network of glands that secrete hormones directly into the bloodstream. These include the pituitary the thyroid the adrenals and the pineal gland, etc.
Endomorph	*See* Somatotypes.
Enzyme	An enzyme is a protein substance that catalyses chemical reactions of various substances without itself being destroyed or altered. Although many enzyme reactions occur within cells, digestive enzymes operate outside the cells in the digestive tract.

Follicle Stimulating Hormone FSH	Secreted by the anterior pituitary gland. Its function in the woman includes the growth of ovarian follicles, oestrogen production, and it is involved in the first portion of the menstrual cycle.
Free Radical	A substance that has lost part of its electrical charge by oxidation. In excess, free radicals can contribute to many illnesses. Free radical sources include air pollution, stress, cigarette smoke, pesticides, burnt foods. Antioxidants reduce the risk of damage from free radicals.
Free T4	Free thyroxine. A blood test that refers to the 'unattached' thyroid hormone that travels in the bloodstream. Every hormone is 'bound' to a protein. The bound hormone is inactive, while the free hormone is active.
Gastrogram	A gastric function test designed to assess gastric acid production (pH), pancreatic enzyme levels and stomach-emptying speed.
Glucagon	A hormone produced by the pancreas that converts glycogen to glucose in the liver. Its secretion is triggered by hypoglycaemia (low blood sugar), and it can be used as a first aid measure for severe hypoglycaemic episodes in people with diabetes.
Glucose Tolerance Factor	A complex comprising chromium, niacin (vitamin B_3) and the amino acids glycine, glutamic acid and cysteine. The GTF is involved in glucose-insulin balance.

Glucose Tolerance Test (GTT)	A two-, five- or six-hour test involving frequent blood glucose measurements after the ingestion of 50–100 gm of soluble glucose. The GTT is used as an aid to the diagnosis of diabetes and hypoglycaemia.
Glycaemic Index (G/I)	A method devised to assess foods according to the extent that certain foods increase the blood sugar. The higher the G/I of food, the speedier the food increases the blood sugar. Many factors influence a food's G/I number, including sugar content and type, and fibre content. The G/I has many inconsistencies, and different lists show differing numbers for the same foods. Generally speaking, the lower the number the better the food for health and weight control. However the G/I listings do not take food quality or nutritional value into account, only a given food's effect on our blood sugar.
Glycogen	The chief carbohydrate stored in animal cells. It is formed from glucose and stored mainly in the liver and muscles. It can be converted back into glucose and released into the circulation when needed.
Haemoglobin (Hb)	A protein-iron compound in the blood which carries oxygen to the cells from the lungs and carbon dioxide away from the cells to the lungs.
Heliobacter Pylori	A bacterial infection that can cause gastritis and stomach ulcers. Usually treated with specific antibiotics.

Hormone Replacement Therapy (HRT)	Replacement of female hormones (oestrogen and/or progesterone). Although chiefly prescribed during and after menopause or hysterectomy, HRT is also prescribed for depression, osteoporosis, arthritis, Alzheimer's disease, low sex drive and pre-menstrual syndrome.
Hydrocortisone	*See* Cortisol.
Hyperinsulinism	Inappropriately high levels of insulin in the blood. Also defined as insulin resistance. Elevated blood insulin leads to calories being converted to fat instead of energy. Hypoglycaemia can also result from insulin excess.
Hyperthyroidism	Hyperactivity of the thyroid gland. This can accelerate all the metabolic processes of the body.
Hypochlorhydria	A deficiency of hydrochloric acid in the stomach's gastric juice.
Hypoglycaemia	Inappropriately low level of blood glucose. Usually caused by adrenal hypofunction or an insulin excess (as in poor diabetes control or hyperinsulinism).
Hypothyroidism	Underactivity of the thyroid gland.
IDDM (Insulin-Dependent Diabetes Mellitus)	Also known as Type I. Thought to be essentially an insulin deficiency caused by a hereditary predisposition.
IgA, IgD, IgE, IgG and IgM	These are all immunoglobulins, which are antibodies that occur in the blood and body secretions and defined according to structure and biological activity. Acute food reactions or allergies are usually associated with an IgE response, and food sensitivities or intolerances are linked to an IgG response.

Insulin Resistance	A term used to define the effects of a typical high-sugar, refined carbohydrate Western diet. The high level of consumed sugar leads to insulin overproduction and fat storage. Many who suffer from late onset diabetes do not have an insulin deficiency but a tendency to be insensitive to the effects of insulin. Their cells do not respond effectively to the insulin message and their blood sugar rises. The blood insulin levels also rise as the body attempts to balance the blood sugar.
Kwashiorkor (Infantile pellagra)	Severe protein deficiency, usually seen in children. Symptoms include retarded growth, skin changes, mental apathy and anaemia. Mainly occurs in tropical climates.
Lactase	A digestive enzyme that converts the sugar in milk (lactose) to glucose and galactose. Lactase deficiency or lactose intolerance is a common condition of infancy. The treatment involves either avoidance of milk products or the use of supplementary lactase prior to eating milk or milk products.
Leaky Gut Syndrome	Increased gut permeability. This can allow the leakage of toxic substances from the gut into the bloodstream. Chronic gut inflammation caused by *Candida albicans* and other parasites can cause a leaky gut.
Lean Body Mass (LBM)	Sometimes termed lean body muscle mass. This is the body mass without the fat component.
Libido	The sex drive or energy.

Luteinizing Hormone (LH)	A hormone, produced by the anterior pituitary that stimulates the secretion of the sex hormones by the ovary and testes. In men, LH induces the secretion of testosterone; in women, LH – working with Follicle Stimulating Hormone (FSH) – stimulates the ovaries to secrete oestrogen.
Lymphatic System	A huge complex of capillaries, valves, duct and nodes, functioning as a waste-disposal system. Toxins can accumulate in the lymph system, and lymphatic drainage techniques using massage can be effective to improve the lymph flow.
Malabsorption	Poor assimilation of nutrients including minerals and fat-soluble vitamins through the gastrointestinal tract or gut. This can occur in many disorders including diarrhoea, gluten sensitivity (coeliac disease), malnutrition, Crohn's disease, after stomach surgery, etc.
Menorrhagia	Abnormally heavy or prolonged menstrual periods. The excessive blood loss can lead to anaemia. (A patient suffering from menorrhagia can lose iron equivalent to 4–6 weeks' dietary iron intake.)
Mesomorph	*See* Somatotypes.
Metabolic Obesity	A term used to describe overweight caused by ill-health.
Myalgic Encephalomyelitis	A chronic illness with symptoms of fatigue, muscle-joint pain, depression and immune deficiency. The term ME is being replaced by Chronic Fatigue Syndrome (CFS). Many doctors consider that ME is

	psychological in origin, and prescribe anti-depressant drugs and stress counselling.
Myxoedema	A severe form of hypothyroidism.
Naturopathy	A treatment system which recognizes that the human body possesses self-curative properties which resist disease. Naturopathic medicine includes many therapies such as hydrotherapy, exercise, nutrition and manipulation. Naturopaths often make use of other auxiliary techniques including acupuncture, homoeopathy and herbalism.
NIDDM (Non-Insulin-Dependent Diabetes Mellitus)	Also termed Type II or late onset diabetes.
Oestrogen	A name for a group of up to 20 different female hormones, the most important being oestrone, oestradial and oestriol. Produced by the ovaries, adrenals and (in men) the testes, it promotes the development of the female secondary sex characteristics and during the menstrual cycle prepares the genital tract for fertilization and conception.
Oestrogen Dominance	A term described by Dr John Lee to define an oestrogen imbalance with a progesterone deficiency. Excessive oestrogen is thought to contribute to fluid retention, overweight, uterine fibroids, endometriosis, ovarian cysts, depression, thyroid imbalance, headaches, raised blood pressure and breast cancer risk.
Omega 3, 6, and 9	The essential fatty acids. The numbers refer to the position of the final double

	bond carbon atoms at the methyl (or 'omega') end of the molecules.
Osteoporosis	Abnormal reduction in bone mass, leading to fractures from slight strain. Causes can include post-menopausal calcium depletion, lack of exercise in the elderly, poor diet, steroid therapy and thyroid or parathyroid disease.
Perimenopause (Premenopause)	The phase before a woman's full menopause, when ovarian hormone production is reducing. Symptoms can begin as early as age 35, and last for up to 15 years. The effects can include depression, muscle-joint problems, fatigue, headaches, insomnia, mood swings, osteoporosis, weight gain and loss of sex drive.
pH	Abbreviation for 'potential hydrogen'. A scale that represents the relative alkalinity or acidity of a solution. Neutral is 7.0, below 7.0 is acid, and above 7.0 is alkaline. The pH value shows the relative concentration of hydrogen atoms in a solution.
Phyto-oestrogens	Plant oestrogens, chiefly found in soya beans. These weak oestrogens are common in Asian and vegetarian diets and are seen by many doctors and health workers as the chief reason for low levels of menstrual and menopausal symptoms in Japanese women.
Pituitary Gland	A vital endocrine gland in the skull, responsible for control of the other endocrine glands such as the adrenals, thyroid, pituitary and ovaries.

PMS (Pre-menstrual Syndrome)	A group of symptoms that occur before menstruation. These can include fluid retention, hypoglycaemia, mood changes and fatigue.
Polycystic Ovary Syndrome (PCOS)	A condition involving hormonal imbalances and insulin resistance. Symptoms caused include excess weight, irregular or non-existent periods, excessive body hair, acne, fatigue and depression. The chief hormonal imbalance involves an excess of Luteinizing Hormone and Follicle Stimulating Hormone, with a resulting high level of oestrogen and testosterone.
Prediabetes	Mild, first-stage diabetes. Usually controlled by diet alone.
Pregnenolone	Sometimes called the 'mother' hormone, because other hormones including DHEA, oestrogen, testosterone, cortisol and progesterone are synthesized from pregnenolone. An adrenal steroid hormone, it is prescribed for depression and rheumatic symptoms.
Probiotics	This term describes the normal, healthy, 'friendly' gut bacteria. The big three are acidophilus, bulgaricus and bifidus. These supplements are used in anti-candida programmes and to generally improve gut health and efficiency.
Progesterone	This hormone is dominant in the second half of a woman's cycle. Suppression of hormonal progesterone production is seen as the cause of oestrogen-dominance symptoms. Natural plant progesterones

are usually prescribed by naturopaths in the form of hypoallergenic moisturizing cream. This is not the same as yam extract.

Prostaglandins (PGs) Hormone-like substances. Over 30 are known. Made by the body from essential fatty acids (EFAs). First isolated from the prostate gland of sheep, PGs are now known to be present in all cells, tissues and organs. The PGs are very short-lived hormone-like chemicals that influence cellular activities. The production of PGs from EFAs requires minerals and vitamins including vitamins B_3 and B_6, vitamin C, zinc and magnesium.

Protomorphogens (Glandular Extracts) The use of animal (usually bovine) glands for treating a variety of illnesses, in use for centuries. The use of such specific tissue has been found beneficial for adrenal, thymus, thyroid, ovarian, pituitary and other gland and organ deficiencies. These 'organ-specific' nutrients provide safe, specific nutritional support to failing or imbalanced glands and organs.

Pulse Test A simple test designed by Dr Arthur F. Coca in 1956. This test is based on the fact that the pulse rate will increase when we eat foods that we are sensitive to and therefore are intolerant of. Many causes of a temporary increase in the pulse rate need to be eliminated first, including stress, exertion, infection and overheating.

Pyridoxine (Vitamin B_6) A member of the vitamin B complex, found in brewer's yeast, rice, wheat germ,

	bran, sunflower seeds, etc. Used to treat fluid retention, PMS, morning sickness in pregnancy, migraine, stress disorders, diabetes, drug and alcohol abuse, and for women on the contraceptive pill or taking oestrogen.
RAST (Radio-Allergo-Sorbent Test)	A test used to demonstrate allergic reactions. It identifies and quantifies IgE in blood that has been mixed with known allergens. Chiefly used in the detection of food allergies.
Raw Glandular Therapy	*See* Protomorphogens.
Raynaud's Phenomenon	Reduced blood flow to the fingers, toes, ears and nose. Symptoms include whiteness followed by cyanosis (bluish discoloration) and pain. Causes include rheumatoid arthritis, Lupus, neck and upper spinal pressure, drug side-effects, malnutrition, hyperthyoidism, injury and high blood pressure. If severe, gangrene can develop.
RDA (Recommended Dietary Allowance)	The amount of nutrients, including proteins, minerals and vitamins, recommended as an essential and necessary part of our daily food and drink intake to maintain normal health. These amounts are based on the 'average' individual needs and do not take into account the requirements of the elderly. The optimal blood and tissue levels, nutritional requirements, biochemical individuality, nutrient and drug interactions and other aspects of physiological function suggest that many

	RDAs for vitamins and minerals and amino acids are too low.
SAD Syndrome (Seasonal Affective Disorder)	A mood disorder triggered by season change. It involves a poor response to light loss during the winter months. Many health workers consider that the pineal gland and the melatonin that is secreted by the pineal gland is the key to SAD treatment and control.
Serotonin (5-hydroxytryptamine)	A naturally occurring derivative of the amino acid tryptophan. It is a neurotransmitter in the brain and also acts as a vaso-constrictor when blood vessels are damaged. Serotonin is a precursor of the hormone melatonin. Prozac and other anti-depressant drugs act by increasing the levels of serotonin.
Somatotypes	A classification of individuals according to body build, based on various physical characteristics. The three primary types are: ectomorph, endomorph and mesomorph. Ectomorphs are slim individuals with highly developed nervous systems and poorly developed digestive systems. Endomorphs are characterized by a soft, rounded frame with a large trunk and thighs and tapering legs. They tend to accumulate fat easily and have a well-developed digestive system. Mesomorphs are predominantly muscular individuals possessing a heavy, hard physique (mainly muscle weight). Mesomorphs tend to gain weight at middle-age.

Syndrome X

A common functional condition involving insulin resistance and elevated blood insulin. This leads to conversion of food (fuel) to body fat instead of energy. The main results of this metabolic switch are as follows:

1   Overweight – often without a diet change
2   PCOS and menstrual problems
3   Raised blood fats
4   A tendency to hypoglycaemia
5   Mild raised blood pressure

Late onset diabetes frequently features in the family history.

Testosterone

A male hormone, produced in the testes. This hormone is essential for the development of the male sexual organs. In women, when raised, it is thought to be one of the causative factors in PCOS and its symptoms. Women with low testosterone levels are prescribed this hormone for loss of libido, migraines, muscle weakness, fatigue and osteoporosis. For men it is prescribed to improve muscle strength, libido, vitality, immune efficiency, glucose metabolism, bone density and strength, and to relieve allergies.

Tinnitus

Noises in the ears including buzzing, ringing, singing, etc. Very common and, when severe, very distressing. Causes can include excessive noise (e.g. pop concerts, personal stereos, etc.), wax in the ears, catarrh, high and low blood pressure, anaemia, vertigo, drug side-effects, bleeding from the ear, Menières disease, ear diseases and cervical disc lesions.

Thyroxine (T4)	The chief thyroid hormone.
Thyroxine Resistance	This term is used to describe a poor conversion of thyroxine (T4) to triiodothyronine (T3), thus explaining the lack of symptom relief that can occur in patients taking replacement T4.
Total T4	A blood test, now considered obsolete, that measures the bound blood thyroxine. The Total T4 has been replaced by the Free T4.
Triglycerides	The principal fat in human blood. It is bound to protein, forming high- and low-density lipoproteins (HDL and LDL). Measuring the total triglycerides and the lipoproteins in the blood offers important clues in the diagnosis of heart disease, diabetes and obesity.
Triiodothyronine (T3)	The most active thyroid hormone metabolized from thyroxine in the peripheral tissue.
TRH (Thyrotropin Releasing Hormone)	A hormone released from the hypothalamus in the brain to stimulate the release of the pituitary hormone thyrotropin (TSH).
TSH (Thyroid Stimulating Hormone)	A pituitary hormone that controls the release of the thyroid hormones. It is measured in the blood to assess thyroid balance.

Uric Acid	A substance in the blood resulting from protein metabolism and excreted through the bladder. When in excess, it forms into crystals, causing gout. An excess of uric acid in the kidneys can give rise to the formation of kidney stones.
Xenobiotics	This is a broad term used to describe a chemical substance foreign to the human metabolism. The xenobiotics include herbicides, pesticides, insecticides, solvents, toxic metals, drugs, food additives, fungicides, alcohols (e.g. ethanol), cocaine, barbiturates, amphetamines and other illegal drugs, organic compounds used in various furnishings and building materials (e.g. formaldehyde).

Resources

THE GENERAL COUNCIL AND REGISTER OF NATUROPATHS
Tel: 01458 840072
Fax: 01458 840075
www.naturopathy.org.uk/members

YORK NUTRITIONAL LABORATORY
Tel: 01904 410410
Fax: 01904 422000
e-mail: ynl@allergy-co.uk
www.allergy-testing.com

BIOLAB MEDICAL UNIT
Tel: 020 7636 5959
Fax: 020 7580 3910
e-mail: lab@biolab.co.uk
www.biolab.demon.co.uk

BIOCARE LTD
Tel: 0121 433 3727
Fax: 0121 433 8705
e-mail: biocare@biocare.co.uk

Nutri Ltd
Tel: 0800 212 742
Fax: 0800 371 731
e-mail: info@nutri.co.uk

Wellspring Trading Ltd ('Serenity Cream')
Tel: 01481 233370
Fax: 01481 235206

The author may be contacted at:
Ridge Cottage
29 Ferncroft Road
Bournemouth
Dorset BH10 6BY
(Please enclose a stamped self-addressed envelope)
e-mail: mlb@martin-budd.com
www.martin-budd.com

References

Chapter 2

E. M. Abrahamson and A. W. Pezet, *Body, Mind and Sugar* (Holt, Rinehart and Winston)

Jennie Brand-Miller *et al.*, *The Glucose Revolution* (Marlow and Co.)

Martin L. Budd, *Diets to Help Diabetes* (Thorsons)

——, *Low Blood Sugar* (Thorsons)

Martin Budd and Maggie Budd, *Recipes for Health – Low Blood Sugar* (Thorsons)

Carlton Fredericks, *Low Blood Sugar and You* (Constellation International)

Fred D. Hofeldt, *Preventing Reactive Hypoglycaemia* (Warren H. Green Inc.)

Gerald Reaven, *Syndrome X* (Simon & Schuster)

Barry Sears, *Enter the Zone* (Regan Books)

John Yudkin, *Pure White and Deadly* (Davis-Poynter)

Chapter 3

Udo Erasmus, *Fats That Heal, Fats That Kill* (Alive Books)
Ann Louise Gittleman, *Eat Fat, Lose Weight* (Keats)
Barry Groves, *Eat Fat, Get Thin* (Vermilion)
Robert E. Kowalski, *Cholesterol and Children* (Thorsons)
Richard Mackarness, *Eat Fat and Grow Slim* (Fontana Books)
Daniel B. Mowrey, *Fat Management* (Victory Publications)
Nigel Plummer, *Dietary Fats and Fatty Acids in Human Healthcare* (Biomed Publications)

Chapter 4

Dr F. Batmanghelidj, *Your Body's Many Cries for Water* (Tagman Press)
Linda Lazarides, *The Waterfall Diet* (Piatkus)
Trevor Smith, *The Side-Effects Book* (Insight Editions)

Chapter 5

Geoffrey Cannon, *Superbug* (Virgin)
Leon Chaitow, *Candida Albicans* (Thorsons)
Leon Chaitow and Natasha Trenev, *Probiotics* (Thorsons)
William G. Crook, *The Yeast Connection* (Professional Books)
John McKenna, *Alternatives to Antibiotics* (Gill and Macmillan)
Orion Truss, *The Missing Diagnosis* (The Missing Diagnosis Inc.)

Chapter 6

Jonathan Brostoff and Linda Gamlin, *The Complete Guide to Food Allergy and Intolerance* (Bloomsbury)

Arthur F. Coca, *The Pulse Test* (Arco Publishing Inc.)

Theron G. Randolph and Ralph W. Moss, *Allergies* (Turnstone Press Ltd)

Mark Varey, Maureen Jenkins and Susan Adams, *Food Sensitivity Guide Book* (York Nutritional Laboratory)

Chapter 7

Jeffrey Bland, *Digestive Enzymes* (Keats)

Susan E. Charmine, *Raw Juice Therapy* (Thorsons)

Edward Howell, *Enzyme Nutrition* (Avery Publishing Group)

Leslie and Susannah Kenton, *Raw Energy* (Book Club Associates)

Chapter 8

D. Lindsey Berkson, *Hormone Deception* (Contemporary Books)

Gillian Ford, *Listening to Your Hormones* (Prima Publishing)

Carlton Fredericks, *Carlton Fredericks Guide to Woman's Nutrition* (Perigee)

William Gelso and Carol Colman, *The Super Hormone Promise* (Pocket Books)

Steven R. Goldstein and Lauri Ashner, *Could It Be Perimenopause?* (Vermilion)

Ellen Grant, *Sexual Chemistry* (Cedar)

Colette Harris and Adam Carey, *PCOS* (Thorsons)

Raquel Martin, John R. Lee and Judi Gerstung, *The Oestrogen Alternative* (Healing Arts Press)

Chapter 9

Ridha Arem, *The Thyroid Solution* (Ballantine Books)

Broda O. Barnes and Lawrence Galton, *Hypothyroidism – The Unsuspected Illness* (Harper & Row)

Martin L. Budd, *Why Am I So Tired?* (Thorsons)

Stephen E. Langer and James F. Scheer, *Solved, The Riddle of Illness* (Keats)

R. McCarrison, *The Thyroid Gland* (Baillière, Tindall and Cox)

M. Sara Rosenthal, *The Thyroid Sourcebook* (Lowell House)

General

Robert C. Atkins, *Dr Atkins Vita-Nutrient Solution* (Simon and Schuster)

Thomas Bartram, *Encyclopaedia of Herbal Medicine* (Grace Publishers)

Jeffrey Bland, *Genetic Nutritioneering* (Keats)

Jeffrey Bland et al., *Clinical Nutrition* (The Institute for Functional Medicine)

Jeffrey Bland (ed), *The Medical Applications of Clinical Nutrition* (Keats)

Eric R. Braverman and Carl L. Pfeiffer, *The Healing Nutrients Within* (Keats)

Leon Chaitow, *Amino Acids in Therapy* (Thorsons)

Michael R. Eades and Mary Dan Eades, *Protein Power* (Thorsons)

Robert Erdmann and Meirion Jones, *The Amino Revolution* (Century)

Marilyn Glenville, *Natural Alternatives to Dieting* (Kyle Cathie Ltd)

Stephen Langer and James Scheer, *How to Win at Weight Loss* (Thorsons)

Kathryn Marsden, *The Complete Book of Food Combining* (Piatkus)

Michael Murray and Joseph Pizzorno, *Encyclopaedia of Natural Medicine* (McDonald Optima)

Roger J. Williams, *Biochemical Individuality* (University of Texas Press)

Index